Belly Dance

Belly Dance:
the dance of mother earth

Tina Hobin

MARION BOYARS
LONDON • NEW YORK

First published in Great Britain and the United States in 2003 by
MARION BOYARS PUBLISHERS LTD
24 Lacy Road, London SW15 1NL

www.marionboyars.co.uk

Distributed in Australia and New Zealand by Peribo Pty Ltd
58 Beaumont Road, Kuring-gai, NSW 2080

10 9 8 7 6 5 4 3 2 1

The Publishers would like to state that this book is an
introduction to the subject, written by a practitioner, and is not a
definitive history. All facts have been checked to the best of our
ability. If you are in any doubt, please check with a medical
expert before practising the belly dance movements.

A CIP catalogue record for this book is available from the
British Library.
A CIP catalog record for this book is available from the Library
of Congress.

ISBN 0-7145-3091-3

Printed in the UK by Bookmarque, London.

CONTENTS

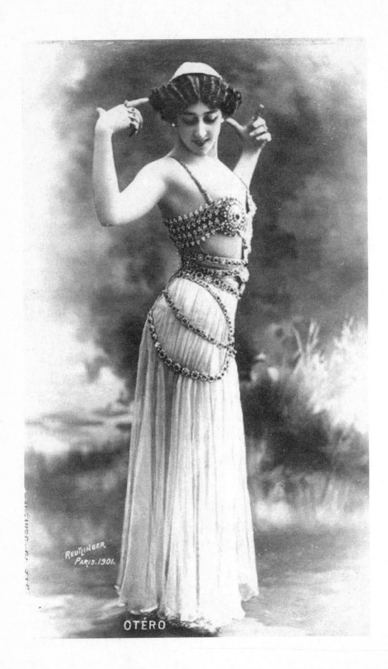

REUTLINGER
PARIS. 1901.

OTÉRO

1

The Origins of Dance

'In the beginning, Eurynome, the Goddess of All Things, rose naked from Chaos, but found nothing substantial for her feet to rest upon, and therefore divided the seas from the sky, dancing lonely upon its waves. She danced towards the south, and the wind set in motion behind her seemed nothing new and apart with which to begin a work of creation. Wheeling about, she caught hold of the north wind, rubbed it between her hands, and behold! the great serpent Ophion. Eurynome danced to warm herself, wildly and more wildly, until Ophion, grown lustful, coiled about those divine limbs and was moved to couple with her. So Eurynome was got with child. Next, she assumed the form of a dove, brooding on the waves, and, in due process of time, laid the Universal Egg. At her bidding, Ophion coiled several times about this egg until it hatched and split in two. Out tumbled all things that exist, her children: sun, moon, planets, stars, the earth with its mountains and rivers, its trees, herbs, and living creatures.' (*The Pelasgian Creation Myth, Greek Myths*, Robert Graves, 1955.)

Throughout history, human beings have used dance to sustain their link with the cosmos and to communicate with their gods as they celebrated the life force and renewal of nature. Evidence tracing the earliest recognisable dance forms back as far as 13000 BCE is provided by the famous cave paintings of Chauvet in France, for example, which depict a sorcerer with arms raised and legs set apart, apparently dancing. Together with more recent depictions, such as the 'Dance of the Goddess' and 'Young God Beside The Tree of Life' from the Mycenaean Ring at the Tholos Tomb of Vapheio 1450 BCE, such evidence enables us to trace the evolution of fledgling dance forms (*The Myth of The Goddess*, Anne Baring and Jules Cashford, 1991). From such representations we can conceive of the basic rhythmic motion used by early practitioners to worship the gods and chart the development of these primitive dance forms into complex mystical, magical and religious cults involving a variety of ceremonies.

Early dance movements were imitative, achieved through the dancers' awareness of their environment and through their observations of the birds and animals around them. By mimicking the characteristic movements of these indigenous species, such as their mating rituals, an imitative dance form was created that forged a rhythmic release of energy through which the dancers displayed an involuntary expression of emotions such as ecstasy and pleasure.

It is easy to visualise how imitative and mimetic dances were performed by our ancestors when basic movements such as leaping, jumping, lunging, squatting and circling are all familiar characteristics of animal behaviour. The uniquely human aspect, however, is that through imitative dance human beings found themselves able to express their joy, grief and physical desires in order to re-live the daily dramas of their lives. Subsequently, over time movements became more complex, varied and rhythmic, creating art forms that Curt Sachs described in his book, *World History of the Dance* (1937), as 'the mother of all arts.'

The various representations of dancing figures found in cave paintings suggest that primitive dance forms played an extremely important role in the social life of our ancestors, who believed that spirits and demons surrounded them and were capable of doing great harm. Without the benefit of science, volcanic eruptions, earthquakes and hurricanes, thunder and lightning, rain, floods and winds, the rising and setting of the sun, the waxing and waning of the moon and even the occurrence of night and day would have remained mysterious. To these ancient people the volatile nature of the cosmos and the natural world was both inexplicable and frightening.

In consequence, humans used magic rites and witchcraft to worship the gods, and, with the help of sorcerers, attempted to appease the angry or hostile gods they believed had caused the catastrophic natural changes they endured. They believed that the gods had inflicted terrible diseases on them, injuries, sickness and hardship that resulted in disability or death. Magicians or medicine men were revered almost universally in early societies as the healers of disease and the leaders of men. In fact, in certain societies where shamanism remains prominent today, in some Inuit and Siberian cultures for example, sorcerers continue to be regarded as the most powerful members of their community (*The Myth of The Goddess*, Anne Baring and Jules Cashford, 1991).

The first dances were an essential part of worship through which human beings felt they were able to establish their relationship with divinity and a unification of the earth with a higher, spiritual world. Through dance they manifested the ethereal sphere of gods, spirits and demons in a form of ritual worship from which it is said religion was born (*Greek Myths*, Robert Graves, 1955).

For our ancient ancestors, nothing equalled the power of dance as a form of ritual worship and magical representation. Dance was also a means of establishing divine intervention, to enable good to be distinguished from evil, and a means of protecting themselves from destructive influences. As the primary concern was the cycle of life, dances were performed ecstatically for all occasions. They celebrated birth, death, rebirth, planting and harvesting, as well as victory in war and a successful hunt. The sacred dance was also a way of evoking the animal soul of humanity, for it was considered vital to maintain a healthy relationship with the unseen powers of life believed to be embodied in the animals surrounding them (*The Myth of The Goddess*, Anne Baring and Jules Cashford, 1991). To this end our ancestors often wore the skins of the animals they had hunted, depending on which animal a ritual focused on. Dance was necessary for initiating the young on reaching puberty and for courtship rituals and fertility rites, which sometimes exploited the hormonal changes induced by lunar activity. C. Knight suggests in his book, *Blood Relations* (1991), it is possible that, 'by using the moon as a clock and by dancing in time with it, palaeolithic women succeeded in keeping in synchrony with one another,' thus regulating menstruation and ovulation. So early dance forms included rain dances, sun and moon worship and supplication to the gods. Dance enabled these humans to enhance the structure and quality of their lives and ritual ceremonies were linked with magical, religious and cultural beliefs.

There is evidence of circle dances and double-circle dances in which the women formed the outer circle and the men the inner circle. In depictions of Stone Age dances from the caves of Tuc D'Aubert and Montespau in South West France, for example, a clear imprint of feet forming a circle have been found. These dances were thought to represent the celestial motion of the moon and the sun and to protect a divine space from intrusion. Spiral dances represented death and rebirth, mimicking the journey of the dead by weaving along a winding path that represented the wandering of the soul.

Circle dances were followed by line dances in which men and women faced each other in rows and repetitively danced towards and then back from one another. In its more recent manifestations the circle dance has altered so that the dancers should not actually take the hand of their fellow dancers but instead link together by holding the corner of a handkerchief (*The World's People and How They Live*, Odhams Press, 1946). This kind of dance is a tradition inherent to the Balkans for example (Jenni Conrad, for the Washington State Arts Commission, 2001) as well as being performed in countries such as Greece and Turkey.

The Cult of the Shaman

Like prehistoric dance, shamanic practice developed as a means of transcending earthly existence and gaining contact with the 'unseen powers' of the spirit world and its many rulers. The historian of religion Mircea Eliade writes, 'It is impossible to imagine a period in which man did not have dreams and waking reveries and did not enter into a 'trance' – a loss of consciousness interpreted as the soul travelling into the beyond,' (*Shamanism: Archaic Techniques of Ecstasy*, Mircea Eliade, 1972). Though the existence of palaeolithic shamans is not irrefutable, the virtually universal assumption that shamanism is associated with hunting supports the belief that it could well be the world's oldest spiritual discipline and medical practice.

The shaman was a kind of sorcerer, a medicine man or man of knowledge, who performed ritual dances in order to gain wisdom of the 'other world' and employ its forces to benefit the inhabitants of this world. The word 'shaman' is thought to have derived from a term employed by the Evenk, a small Tungus-speaking group of hunters and reindeer herders in Siberia, meaning a priest with healing powers who could influence the spirits to bring about good and evil. Shamanism is not a single unified religion, however, but more a cross-cultural form of religious practice that manifests itself in many different forms.

The cult was widespread among the hunter cultures of Africa, in parts of North Western Australia, Northern Asia, among the Inuit and also the Lapps of Northern Scandinavia (*Primitive Man*, Andreas Lommel, 1966). Shamanism was also of vital importance to the Native Americans of the Pacific Coast, among the Indian tribes of the South East, and the North East Woodlands and to other North American tribes such as the Zuni, Hopi and Plains Tribes. Ethnologists and anthropologists, including Mircea Eliade, believe it is likely that shamanism has been practised worldwide for thousands of years and that it has remained remarkably consistent in technique despite varying cultural diversities. Today in many parts of the world, the arts of healing and trance are still practised by shamans. Eliade's research, for example, draws many parallels between the palaeolithic shamanic rituals and those practised in modern day Siberia. As well as the ancient rituals beings preserved in contemporary shamanic practices of the Arctic, Borneo and Amazonian cultures, the spread of New Age culture has promoted shamanism across the globe. In New Age culture, the term retains the same reference point: a shaman is someone who is thought to be in contact with the spirits (*The Shaman*, Piers Vitebsky, 1995).

Although there were some female shamans, such as those of the Kung Bushman tribes of the Kalahari Desert in Botswana (*Evolution of Shamanism*, Gina Scott, for the International Conference on the Study of Shamanism, 2002), shamans were predominantly men. The shaman, who was also known as the witch doctor, was usually chosen because of his extra sensory powers and psychic predisposition (*Shamanism Today*, Turner 1972, from www.shamanism.today) although sometimes the role was inherited. As many shamans were believed capable of exerting immense transcendental power, either for good or for evil, they were generally feared in their communities. When ordered by members of the tribe to carry out certain functions, if successful, they would gain further prestige within the community.

A shaman would act primarily as a priest and physician, and his mission was to mediate between members of the tribal community and operate as their ancestors' spokesman, controlling the elements, operating as a prophet and healing the sick by exorcising evil spirits who threatened their well being. It was often believed that illness was caused by evil spirits that entered the body of their own accord, or by the absence of a soul, which the shaman would pursue and charm back into the body by performing a divine service of magic incantation and ritual dance (*The Shaman*, Piers Vitebsky,1995).

In certain shamanic cultures, such as the San Tribe of South Africa, the sick were, and still are in some places, placed in the centre of a circle and danced around until the evil spirit was exorcised. This magic ritual can last for several hours. It was important for the shaman to acquire guardian spirits with whom he communicated and maintained contact through ecstatic dancing and incantations, during which he would enter a trance-like state and assume the form of an animal or spirit of the dead. In most shamanic practices, herbal remedies were also used to help cure the sick. These early methods of medical practice were essentially magical, an art of sorcery from which it is said the origins of the medical profession and priesthood were derived.

Dance was central to early shamanism. It was used to induce a trance-like state along with rhythmic chanting, hand clapping and various other techniques, including hyperventilating and the ingestion of hallucinatory drugs. During his altered state of consciousness, the shaman would enter into a trance within which he would hallucinate and his whole body tremble.

Sometimes he would double over as if in excruciating pain and would have to be supported by other members of the tribe. In some cases, sickness and pain were considered to be a vital part of the basic shamanic experience. The Hungarian explorer Vilmos Diószegi collected many reports from Siberia of shamanic vocations being chosen for prospective shamans by the 'black spirits' that made them ill and forced them to take up shamanism to escape suffering (*Dreamtime and Inner Space*, Holger Kalweit, 1984).

Convulsive dances were prevalent in shamanic cultures and were dominated by the men of the tribe. They would dance ecstatically with tremendous energy, convulsively stamping their feet, hopping from one foot to the other and wildly jumping and leaping around in circles to rhythmic chants, hand claps and the beat of drums, rattles or tambourines. The shaman would invoke through dance the state of altered consciousness that enabled him to make contact with the spirit world. Shamanic technique may involve anything that disrupts everyday psychological processes to produce a new rhythmic pattern and dance is believed to aid this restructuring of our consciousness (*Dreamtime and Inner Space*, Holger Kalweit, 1984).

During their religious ceremonies, the aim of the chief dancers was therefore to lose complete control at the climax of the performance and enter into an altered state of mind. To prevent any of the dancers from harming themselves whilst in this state of uncontrollable frenzy, they were often tethered by four ropes held by assistants.

Dancing for the Hunt

Early humans depended on animals for their survival. They hunted animals such as bison, deer, zebra, horses, bears, mammoths and rhinoceroses for food, clothing, weapons and other artefacts. It has been supposed that animals were plentiful and easy game in ancient times but it is more than likely that hunters were not always successful in their pursuit. To ensure the successful outcome of hunting expeditions, it was considered essential for the shaman to identify with the animal he represented. By wearing an animal skin, a mask and by mimicking the animal's ways he could reinforce and increase the power of magic over the animal's soul. A shaman believed that in these magic hunting rituals he became the animal's spirit, which he controlled through the ecstasy of the dance.

Scenes connected with magic rites relating to hunting cultures have been discovered in cave painting and rock engravings in the Lascaux Cave in South West France 15000 BCE which, with its extensive chambers and passageways, contains the most famous examples of colourful prehistoric rock art of large animals ever to be found from the Upper Palaeolithic Period.

In the entrance of a palaeolithic cave in the Dordogne in Laussel, France, our ancestors carved a nude image of the great mother, 'Venus' 22000-18000 BCE. Her pendulous breasts, bulging belly and pubic triangle are well defined, suggesting pregnancy. Her left hand points towards her large belly and the other hand holds a bison or lunar horn, painted in red ochre, which has been interpreted as the moon. There is dispute over the exact meaning of the notches carved on the horn but they are thought to relate to the thirteen days of the waxing moon and the thirteen months of the lunar year. The position of her body, which draws a curve between the waxing of the moon and the fecundity of the womb, suggests that the figurine was intended to highlight the relationship between the heavenly and earthly orders (*The Myth of The Goddess*, Anne Baring and Jules Cashford, 1991). Over time the figure of Venus also came to be associated with 'myths of the mistress of the beasts', a goddess with influence over animals who drives them towards the hunters during the chase.

Cave paintings at Altamira in Northern Spain dating from around 13000 BCE (*Altamira*, Deutches Museum, Munchen 2003) as well as in other regions of the world, illustrate what appears to be a shaman wearing antlers masquerading as an animal. The shaman dances ecstatically with arms raised, pictured together with numerous large animals such as rhinoceroses, bulls, bears, horses, zebras, deer and various hunting scenes. The 'Animal–shaman' at the renowned Trois Frères caves in Northern France 14000 BCE illustrates a sorcerer dancing above a group of wild beasts, and in the centre a shaman, dressed as a bison, dances holding a hunting bow (*The Myth of The Goddess*, Anne Baring and Jules Cashford, 1991).

Cybele, the Greek goddess Artemis, Hathor and Isis were often associated with domestic and wild animals, particularly those hunted, for as mistresses of animals they were responsible for the hunt (*Secrets of the Stone Age*, Richard Rudgely, 2000). The myth of the mother goddess is linked to familiar figures from the art of Old Europe, such as the goddess of the animals. One seal from the tomb of Thassos in Crete 15000 BCE depicts a goddess on a mountain top with lions and other followers engaged in worship.

Traces of the palaeolithic 'Hunt Goddess,' such as that depicted in the statuette Venus of Willendorf (24000-22000 BCE) have been discovered wherever ancient people existed and her magic associations with animals have been found throughout the world. The hunt goddess was a subsidiary of the mother goddess myth whose associations with weaponry may be considered to be in opposition with the nurturing role of the mother but who developed from this myth nonetheless. Some argue that the mother goddess myth may include the hunter but the hunter story cannot easily encompass the mother (*On the Road of the Winds: An Archaeological History of the Pacific Islands*, Professor Patrick Kirch, 2000). In more recent times among the Kalahari Bushmen, as dawn rises on the day of the hunt, a female shaman performs a ritual dance through which she communicates with the spirits of the beasts. It is believed by the bushmen that the spirits indicate the animals are about to die of their own volition to feed the people of the tribe.

Although hunt dancers were not often women, images of sacred women standing with arms raised, together with some whose arms are supported by smaller male figures standing on either side of them, have been found in stone cave paintings. Among the examples of depictions of female hunt dancers are the Stone Age cliff paintings found by Mary Leaky in Central Tanzania, in which the hunt dancers are almost always women. During the hunt it was a function of the women to adopt this stance, with arms raised, acting as recipients of cosmic energy. A further example of a female hunt dance is provided by the Kalahari bushmen today, as a Kalahari shaman woman performs a special dance at dawn on the day of the hunt, invoking the protective Dawn Star (Venus) who is called the hunter, and communing with the spirits of the animals who will voluntarily die to feed humans. (*The Great Cosmic Mother* by Monica Sjoo and Barbara Mor, 1991.)

Sacrificial and Trance Dances

Mimetic and imitative forms of dance varied greatly in style, from the exhilarating frenzied movements of the shamanic or medicine dance to the acrobatic dance that so impressed and amused the Egyptians, and the more gentle movements of the rain dance. Nevertheless, gentle though the rain dances might have been, they may well have ended with a violent act.

During the rain dances of the Pacific Islands and the West Indies, in which women danced naked, it was not uncommon for a young woman to be sacrificed 'to the blood-thirsty God Oro,' (*On the Road of the Winds: An Archaeological History of the Pacific Islands*, Professor Patrick Kirch, 2000).

Although human sacrifice seems to us to be barbaric, such ancient sacrificial rites of humans are believed to have kept tribes together. The Aztecs, for example, are amongst those ancient civilisations who are supposed to have fed their gods with human hearts and blood (*Cannibalism and Human Sacrifice*, Gary Hogg, 1966).

The Macumba is a form of voodoo mainly practiced by Brazilians, developed from a religion of African origin. Macumba is an umbrella term used for the two principle forms of African spirit worship: Candomble and Umbanda. It originated from the shipping of black slaves to Brazil in the 1550s. Macumba rituals are usually held in isolated areas of the Amazon jungle and at night on the infamous Copacabana beach. The Copacabana festival is a combination of African religion and magical cults, the worship of pagan gods and catholic saints with whom they are associated. Yemanja, the African sea goddess who is also likened to the Virgin Mary and is the main focus of worship, was brought to Brazil by Yoruba slaves from the region of Africa now known as Nigeria. The worshippers mainly dress in white, a colour favoured by the goddess Yemanja, and they carry candles, which are set in pre-prepared holes, as well as gifts which are offered in honour of Yamanja to the sea. During the Macumba rituals worshippers become possessed by gods and demons in the hope of obtaining power to acquire authority, wealth and love, or the ability to reap terrible revenge upon their enemies (*Marvels and Mysteries, Rituals and Magic*, Parragon Press, 1997).

As the Macumba celebrations progress, the charged atmosphere and pulsating rhythms of the drums encourage participants to take part in frenzied, almost orgiastic dancing until entering a near hypnotic state. Towards the climax of the evening, as the high priest summons down the gods, one by one the dancers cease dancing and prostrate themselves.

'The Ghost Dance' is a dance of the Sioux and other American Indians (*The Ghost-Dance Religion and the Sioux Outbreak of 1890*, James Mooney, 1992). Here dancers move monotonously around and around in circles until every dancer has collapsed on to the ground in what appears to be a seizure. In the late 19th century 'The Ghost Dance' was performed by the Sioux in a desperate bid to rid their land of hostile white invaders. North Mexican tribes took part in dances on altars, also whirling around until similarly delirious and frothing at the mouth, destroying the altars in their uncontrollable madness, before falling unconscious.

In Bali, young men have traditionally taken part in a religious dance called the Kris, based on the idealistic thought of the Rwa Bhineda doctrine (*Bali Music and Dance*, www.kecak.com, 2003). Kris always took place at night by torchlight and was conceived as a frenzied hypnotic dance of good and evil, in which the dancers frequently inflicted terrible wounds upon themselves (*The World's People and How They Live*, Odhams Press, 1946). As a result, dancers were often prevented from using real weaponry to avoid harming other participants. The dance is named after the traditional sword used in Barong plays and tells the story of Balinese men who used the Kris to battle with Rangda, the demon queen. Rangda, however, put the men into a trance-like state of unconsciousness. When they came to, they were so distressed by their failure to overcome her that they tried to impale themselves on their swords, the Kris. Fortunately for them, their trance states would prevent them from being injured.

The Earth Mother and Ancient Cultures

It is believed that belly dance may be one of the oldest dance forms and that it developed from the fertility dances of the mother goddess cult. Its origins are closely linked to fertility and childbirth rituals which, through time, because of the influence of many different countries and cultures, evolved in many different forms.

From the earliest cultures of the Palaeolithic Era (around 50000-10000 BCE) to the Neolithic Era (which is a phrase used to combine the New Stone Age of around 10000 – 5500 BCE with the Copper Age of 5500-3500 BCE) there is evidence that various forms of sacred dance and ritual fertility dances linked to the earth mother goddess evolved.

For example, there is evidence from pre-dynastic graves in Egypt of a widespread cult of the mother goddess, Neith or Nit, who was usually shown wearing her emblem shield crossed with two arrows, linking her to the hunt goddess myth, weaponry and warfare. On occasion, though this is extremely rare, Neith and other such female figurines represented the goddess as a cow, and many such figurines are considered to have been votive offerings to beg for fertility or rebirth in the after life. In his book, *The Inner Reaches of Outer Space: Metaphor as Myth and as Religion* (1986), Joseph Campbell points out that woman, 'as the mother of life and nourisher of life was thought to assist the earth symbolically in its productivity,' and is depicted as such in neolithic pottery. Because in giving birth the woman's body performs an act of creation it is linked to the mysteries of nature's evolution and the creation of the earth.

In early societies, it was thought that women possessed magical powers. It was believed that their fertility and that of the earth on which they toiled created food for everyone.

Though it was unusual for women to take part in animal, magic or hunting dances, they were usually the only participants in fertility rituals which consisted of birth dances, the consecration of young women, mourning rituals, sun and moon worship, rain and harvest dances.

To our ancestors, as the earth mother was the nourisher and preserver of the universe, she represented nature, productiveness and childbirth and became a symbol of life, death and rebirth, celebrated through sacred dance, music and singing. To ancient civilisations, goddesses manifested themselves in everything around them: in the waters, wind, mountains, trees and vegetation, and in the sky, sun, moon and stars. They were also associated with animals, both wild and domestic, particularly birds and snakes whose shapes they could adopt.

In ancient times, breasts were sacred and treated with great reverence. Fertility statuettes of goddesses cupping their breasts in their hands symbolically flowing with milk, and of a mother suckling a child at her breast, were a reminder to our ancient ancestors of the goddesses' ability to nurture, provide sustenance and maintain the balance of life. According to the Greeks, the original shape of a bowl was formed from the breasts of Helen of Troy (*Goddess Mother of Living Nature*, Adele Getty, 1990). The females of the Zuni tribe in North America still make pottery in the shape of breasts.

Based on numerous sacred images and fertility figures discovered deriving from the Neolithic Period, it is thought that magic rites and fertility cults became prominent. In early civilisations the sacred nuptial union of a king and queen represented the deities and ensured the fertility of the land. These great occasions were celebrated with pomp and ceremony, lavish feasts, dancing and singing.

There are many examples of fertility dances that were practised, in particular the phallic dances performed by the Altia Turks and tribes in Corbeau, North Western Brazil. These dancers, who were usually women, had large phalluses made of bast, a wood fibre, and testicles made of red cones picked from the trees which they held close to their bodies with both hands. Dancing one behind the other while leaning forward and stamping their right foot in double quick time, they would suddenly leap wildly along with ferocious coitus movements while groaning loudly, provoking their female partners who would playfully disperse, laughing and shrieking.

Shrines and countless images of goddess figures in their many forms and with a multitude of names have been discovered in almost every culture around the world. How this cult spread so far and wide is not clear. The abundance of these sacred images testifies to the obsession with fertility, religious imagination and the veneration of life and worship of the great earth mother among ancient civilisations.

Ritual Dances of the Pygmy

Pygmies are renowned for taking a great delight in dancing. Their ecstatic war, rain and animal dances, which have survived for thousands of years, include a great variety of movements, each varying in style from tribe to tribe and region to region. Only the female pygmies of Central Africa and Australia teach their children to dance from an early age as part of their tribal culture.

The African Pygmies were particularly skilled at dancing. From as early as the 3rd millennium BCE, the Egyptians recognised their tremendous artistic talents, in particular their acrobatic skills, and brought them to Egypt to entertain, service their gods and dance in religious processions. Anyone who actually presented a dancing pygmy to a king as a gift was held in the highest esteem.

During the reign of Neferkare, 5th King of the 6th Dynasty

who lived from 2246 BCE to 2152 BCE, a caravan master named Harkhuf, who was also a learned priest, made many expeditions into Lower Nubia, Southern Egypt. On one of them he found and brought back a trained dancing pygmy from the Sudan and on his return wrote immediately to the court informing the new boy pharaoh of the pygmy. The pharaoh promptly dictated a letter to Harkhuf, asking him to bring the pygmy to the palace of Memphis at once. The royal letter written by the pharaoh is said to be one of the most remarkable documents remaining from the ancient world. Harkhuf was so touched by the letter he had it inscribed on the façade of one particular tomb so that everyone could read in future the following:

'I have noted the contents of your letter which you sent to me, the King, at the palace, in order that I might know that you returned in safety from Yam with the troops that were with you. You have said in your letter that you have brought numerous rich beautiful gifts, which the goddess Hathor, Lady of Imu (said to be part of Yam), has granted to me, the King of Upper and Lower Egypt, Neferkare, who lives forever and ever. You have also said in your letter that you have brought me back from the Land of Ghosts [unknown regions south of Egypt] a pygmy of [the kind employed therein] that dances for [their] god, like the pygmy which the keeper of the Sacred Treasure, Burded brought back from Punt in the time of King Isesi. You have said to your majesty: Never before has one like him been brought by any other who has reached Yam,' (*Ancient Records of Egypt,* James Henry Breasted, 1906).

There are other historical accounts that include references to pygmy tribes. Curt Sachs, in *World History of the Dance,* (1937), describes the rolling of the pelvis and movements of the rectus abdomini practised by the pygmies of Uganda as being especially significant. The dance emphasised the abdomen as the seat of all sexual and child bearing activity. The original aim of the magical coital movements was to promote life and growth.

'They sat on the ground and rhythmically struck it with their thighs and, or, elbows, while simultaneously turning themselves around on their bottoms, rolling their heads, swinging their tiny bellies around and rocking their bodies to and fro.'

Tribes of North Western Brazil and North Africa were also well known for their movements of the rectus abdomini and the trembling, quivering, undulating movements of their bodies (*World History of the Dance*, Curt Sachs, 1937). These dances also included intricate movements of the muscles in their backs and breasts, very similar to the feats performed by female dancers in Egypt several centuries ago.

The rolling and rotating movements of the pelvis and abdomen, as performed by pygmies and other tribal communities in fertility and magic dances, are amongst the oldest dance movements of which we have a written account. They relate to what travellers began to describe as the hip dance, posterior dance or belly dance. Many of these movements are still being practised in the Near East, Middle East, North Africa and the West.

In Loango on the West Coast of Africa, the purpose of the pelvic dance was thought to be ancestor worship of past generations and a means of glorifying the transmission of life to those yet to be born. In Cambodia and East Africa, tribal dance consisted of vibrant, trembling, undulating and snake-like movements of the body. Natives from the Celebes in Indonesia adopted the abdominal dance from the Egyptians. It was known as Masseri or Messer, an Arabic word meaning Egyptian.

There are isolated examples of abdominal dances existing in the South Seas, for example in New Guinea, Hawaii, Eastern Polynesia and Central Africa where the dance is a means of sexual selection.

Dances of Ancient Egypt

In ancient times religious experiences were often physical and expressed mainly through dance which became a sacrificial rite. Childbirth and fertility rituals, orgiastic rites and magic dances were an integral part of religious ceremonies.

Many ancient religions are thought to originate in Ancient Egypt. Before examining these in more detail and in order to understand the development of dance, we should remind ourselves here of the chronology of Dynastic Egypt.

The two ancient kingdoms of Upper and Lower Egypt, whose origins date from around 3000 BCE, were first unified following the conquest of the North by Menes, the King of Upper Egypt (although the fertile river Nile flood plain had supported the agriculture of tribal settlements from a much earlier date). Ruling from Memphis, establishing himself as the first king of the first Pharaonic Dynasty in the Nile Delta, Menes rule lasted until 2884 BCE.

As contemporary historical records began to be translated, including ancient king-lists, dated inscriptions and astronomical records, a number of major divisions of time emerged.

Though there is dispute over the exact dates for each period, for the purposes of this account I will use these standard dates as provided by the Oxford University Press (*The Oxford History of Ancient Egypt*, Ian Shaw, 2000). The divisions are as follows (see over):

Pre-dynastic Period	5300-3000 BCE
Early Dynastic Period (1st-2nd Dynasty)	3000-2686 BCE
The Old Kingdom (3rd-8th Dynasty)	2686-2160 BCE
1st Intermediate Period (9th-10th Dynasty	2160-2055 BCE
Middle Kingdom (11th-14th Dynasty)	2055-1650 BCE
2nd Intermediate Period (15th-17th Dynasty)	1650-1550 BCE
New Kingdom (18th-20th Dynasty)	1550-1069 BCE
3rd Intermediate Period (21st-25th Dynasty)	1069-664 BCE
Late Period (26th-30th Dynasty)	664-332 BCE
Ptolemaic Period (Macedonian-Ptolemaic Dynasty)	332-30 BCE
Roman Period	30 BCE-395 CE

There will also be reference to the Pharaonic Period, a phrase which historians use to mean the period spanning over 3000 years, beginning when the Egyptian kings or pharaohs first started to rule in Egypt in 3000 BCE and lasting up to 664 BCE (*The Oxford History of Ancient Egypt,* Ian Shaw, 2000). However, as by the end of the New Kingdom in 1069 BCE, the Egyptians' greatest achievements were behind them, it is up to this period which mostly concerns us.

A pharaoh (an ancient Egyptian word meaning 'great house') was a titled ruler, a king or queen of Ancient Egypt, a representative of the gods and also the living son or daughter of the chief god Ra. Ancient Egyptians believed their king or queen was a god with great magical powers. Their gods and goddesses were recognised in various forms, some being represented in human form, others in the shape of animals, and still others in half human, half animal form. The pharaoh was at the pinnacle of Egyptian society. Beneath him, in descending order, were the noblemen, priests, officials, scribes, artisans, unskilled labourers, farmers and peasants. The small but elite group at the top was endowed with wealth and authority. A much larger group below the elite was comprised mainly of administrators.

Tradition and pictorial representation in art suggest that Egyptian women enjoyed a status not shared with women of other civilisations. Paintings of court life show ladies with their consorts in relaxed and intimate mood, but also with a dignity suggestive of independence. Ancient Egyptian women of rank could own property, they enjoyed legal rights and they were often literate (there is an Egyptian word for female scribe). It should also be remembered that the inheritance of the pharaonic line was only achieved through marriage to female offspring of the Royal House, and for this reason, brothers married sisters to gain the throne. The Egyptian pantheon was imbued with femininity, principally through the cult of Isis, all important mother goddess (and of nature and fertility), as through her, together with Osiris, the continuing cycle of regeneration through birth and death became possible.

In fact, Egypt is placed by many historians as the most renowned country in the world for its religion and worship of numerous deities who played an extremely important role in their lives. To begin with, every settlement and town in Ancient Egypt had its own god and goddesses, many of whom were elevated to state gods by pharaohs and priests in dynastic times to become universal cult gods and goddesses symbolising empowerment and unification.

The first gods that the Ancient Egyptians worshipped were male and female deities in the form of animals and later in a form that was part human, part animal. In the Old Kingdom (2686-2160 BCE) Re of Heliopolis was state god, in the New Kingdom (1550-1069 BCE) following in time was Amun of Thebes. Also worshipped as universal deities were the gods Atum of Heliopolis, Ptah of Memphis and Horus of Edfu (*Women of Ancient Egypt*, Barbara Watterson, 1998).

Ancient Egyptians believed that gods such as Atum, Hathor, Isis, Nut and Geb were originally responsible for the creation of the cosmos, our world, and all living things, as well as birth and rebirth. In honour of these important gods and goddesses, they built temples and statues, which ultimately led to the creation of a unique, but very complex, religious culture that survived for over 3000 years.

Atum, the father of the gods, was a self-created deity, who emerged from a fathomless watery pit to be the first entity to appear before creation. Atum was the creator god, who created all things, including humanity, from his own being. Usually he was represented in human form, wearing a double crown of the two kings of Upper and Lower Egypt and he was worshipped at Heliopolis where he was later united with Re to become a sun god - known as Re-Atum. Atum mated with himself and produced Shu, the god of air, and Tefnut, the goddess of moisture, who were the parents of Geb, the earth god and Nut, the sky goddess. Geb and Nut became lovers and consequently gave birth to Osiris and his wife Isis, her sister Nephthys and her husband Seth. Atum was the great god of providence, whose radiant light established his supremacy over the great River Nile to ensure the fertility of the soil, so that it would continue to provide and produce sustenance.

Hathor was the cow goddess of Dendera, in whose honour the beautiful temple of Dendera was built during the 12th Dynasty of the Middle Kingdom 1985-1773 BCE (*Religion and Magic in Ancient Egypt*, Rosalie David, 2002.) She was shown either in the shape of a cow, or in the form of a woman, wearing upon her head a crown of cow's horns with a solar disc between them. Hathor was a fertility goddess who was called upon to assist at the birth of a child. She was often depicted suckling the infant pharaohs. She was a protector of women in childbirth, patron of motherhood, mistress of music, song and dance, goddess of love, peace and wisdom, and was worshipped as a funerary goddess. Although the role was not always well-defined, the cult of the cow goddess extended beyond the boundaries of Egypt.

Many of the images found in houses and in shrines dedicated to Hathor and other Egyptian goddesses were described as either dolls or concubine figurines for the deceased. They were placed in the graves of men, women and children in tombs, possibly by the tomb owners themselves before they died, for their use in the afterlife (*Religion and Magic in Ancient Egypt*, Rosalie David, 2002).

The greatest goddess of Ancient Egypt, and divine ruler of the country, was Isis, the goddess of magic and protector of power against evil. She was usually depicted in human form. As the mother of all gods, she acquired many names and was closely associated with other Egyptian goddesses in her numerous and diverse roles. Isis married her brother Osiris, who introduced religion and law and taught the Ancient Egyptians how to cultivate their land. Because Isis was closely associated with the cow goddess Hathor, she was also often portrayed wearing a crown comprising solar disc and cow's horns. Isis was believed to have discovered wheat and barley, and taught her people how to make bread. She was also associated with marriage and through her magic was able to cure diseases. To the Greeks she was a corn goddess and the deity who gave birth to nature.

Isis's husband Osiris was the most important god of all. He was the god of fertility and of resurrection in the other world. Osiris was supposed to have taught the Egyptian people how to till and cultivate the land and introduced them to religion and law. He was led to a cruel death by his jealous and evil brother Seth, who chopped up his body and scattered the pieces far and wide so that they would never be found. But Isis, his loving, dutiful and distraught wife, sought and gathered the dismembered parts of his body, pieced them together and bound them in bandages. She then breathed life into him, giving him mortality and rebirth. He then became the god of the underworld. Isis greatly mourned the death of her beloved husband and her tears that flowed endlessly were said to have flooded many parts of the Nile. It was not until the death of her husband Osiris that she conceived her son Horus by using her exceptional magical powers.

Horus the Falcon eventually revenged his father's terrible death by castrating Seth and becoming King of Egypt. He became the principal god of Egyptian religion and was associated with many other deities. One of his functions was funerary and involved being a protector of canopic jars, which contained the lungs or other organs removed from the deceased during the rituals of embalming. So the four demi-gods who assisted the goddesses, Isis, Nephthys, Neith and Serket in protecting these canopic jars were known as the 'Four Sons of Horus' (*Religion and Magic in Ancient Egypt*, Rosalie David, 2002).

The oldest magical religious texts inscribed in hieroglyphics were discovered on the walls of passageways and in chambers in the pyramids of Saqqara from the 5th Dynasty onwards. Numerous religious texts were also found on the walls of tombs of the Middle Kingdom (2055-1650 BCE) and New Kingdom (1550-1069 BCE). Evidence found elsewhere suggests that these magic rites, religious cults and rituals that originated in Egypt spread to many other regions of the world.

Although in name the king was the sole priest in each of Egypt's temples, in practice, the duties of administering to the gods needs on a daily basis were delegated to those priests described as 'servants of god' or 'hm-ntr'. During the reign of Herodotus and by the time that the New Kingdom had emerged there was a permanent class of 'lay-priests' whose purification requirements included ritual bathing and cleansing of the mouth along with shaving the head.

They were expected to satisfy their gods by providing them

with nourishment, music, dancing, and spiritual sustenance from which they were supposed to have derived much pleasure. The ranks and duties of the priests varied greatly. Some were employed as bearers of shrines in religious ceremonies and processions or as sacred scribes, judges, administrators and state officials. The most honoured position was that of the chief of priests. Priests fervently believed in astronomy and astrology; many were prophets and wise men acting as advisers and counsellors for the pharaoh. They were also responsible for the burial of the dead, supervised mummification of the deceased and assisted in funerary ceremonies.

Male priests either inherited their priesthood from their fathers or were enlisted as priests by the pharaoh from the ranks of the educated elite. They wore leopard skins over the linen robes, similar to the robes worn by the pharaohs on special occasions. Illustrations show that the linen garments worn by priests varied considerably in style. Sometimes they are pictured wearing a circular cloak or a tight tunic, or draped in linen skirts with a brace over one shoulder, sometimes with a wide sash added around the hips. During the 1st Dynasty, the king performed on grand occasions, often dancing before his god. Any man who knew how to perform 'The Dance of the Gods' was highly honoured and protected. A scene from the great stone, Head of Narmer, discovered at Hieraconpolis, is thought to be that of the dance of the gods. Here, King Narmer and his queen are seated in a shrine and behind the queen are what appear to be dancing men. Sometimes the king danced at Dendera in the temple of Hathor where he was greeted by chanting.

The Cult of the Earth Mother

Around the world our ancient ancestors believed that caves

were the womb of the great earth mother and that to go into a cave was to enter into her deep mystical secrets. Caverns and caves were the principal places in which the goddesses were worshipped and in which female initiation and religious rites were practised. The Minoan cave shrines of Ida and Eileithyia, the goddess of childbirth and motherhood, provided a holy sanctuary for women seeking protection and solace and were divine birthplaces for the gods and mothers-to-be. Some large caves and caverns were found to have contained altars and others became religious centres of learning.

The worship of the mother goddess was possibly the most complex cult of all. It greatly influenced the development of ancient religions and become one of the oldest established surviving religions of the ancient world. The purpose of fertility worship was to ensure the fertility of the earth and the continuation of human beings. The mother goddess cult developed between the 3rd and 5th millennium BCE in an area of fertile land between Israel and the Persian Gulf that stretched to Western Asia, the Indus Valley and Aegean Crete. Eventually the cult extended far and wide from the Iberian Peninsula to Central and North West Europe.

From both the Palaeolithic Era and the Neolithic Era, numerous statuettes of the female form in the upright or squatting positions adopted for childbirth have been discovered by archaeologists in different continents. The earliest examples from Egypt are those of the Neolithic Period. These images were either sculpted from clay, stone, bone, ivory, faience (glazed earthenware) or carved from wood. Each depicted women with rounded buttocks and broad hips, large and heavy breasts, prominent bellies and genitalia, symbolising the functions of motherhood, fertility, regeneration and abundance.

Many of these fertility images were picked out with numerous dots. Others, such as those found in New Guinea, had features emphasised by being painted in red ochre. This is thought likely to have represented the blood of a woman's monthly cycle and blood shed during childbirth.

Neolithic examples of squatting figures used as cult images have been discovered on rock paintings in many countries, including California, New Zealand's South Island and Australia.

When the Greeks reached the Aegean, they found the Aegeans worshipped the great mother goddess and learned to honour her too. They called her Demeter, 'Goddess of the Harvest', meaning corn or barley mother, and she became the greatest goddess in Ancient Greece. Every year, crowds of men and women travelled from all over the Hellenic and Roman world to attend the ceremony of 'The Greater Mysteries' at the great temple of Eleusis, a shrine for the divinity. Here they celebrated the myth of Persephone, daughter of Demeter, who was taken into the underworld by Hades to be his bride. When her daughter was taken from her, Demeter vowed that no seed would grow again and that she would keep all seeds hidden in the earth. She would not set foot on Olympus until her daughter was restored to her and corn would not sprout until she returned. Hades let Persephone return, but by tricking her into eating the seed of a pomegranate he ensured she would return to him for part of the year. Once Persephone rejoined her mother, Demeter transformed the entire plain of Eleusis into a sea of corn.

The ancient Eleusian rite was always held in the open air and was the most important Greek agricultural festival. Originally, it was a mother earth fertility ritual that became one of the universal cults of Ancient Greece. The annual mysteries of Eleusis were the most revered sacred rites celebrated through dance in honour of Persephone, Demeter and Dionysus, the divine child. Those who were initiated into the mysteries of Eleusis, which originated on the island of Crete, never dared divulge their secrets, so knowledge of the final rites was lost.

The cult of Cybele, a great Asiatic fertility goddess emanating from Phrygia and one of the many personifications of the great earth mother, was celebrated by her 'corybants', priests of Cybele, whose orgiastic rites were always accompanied by loud music, screeching and ecstatic dancing. The Emperor Claudius, whose date of birth is officially 1st August 10 BCE, celebrated the spring festival of the sacred tree in Rome and with it the orgiastic rites of Attis, son, but also lover, of Cybele (*Greek Myths*, Robert Graves, 1955). Each year on the 22nd of March, a pine tree was cut and brought to the sanctuary of Cybele, where it was treated as a great divinity. It was covered in woollen bands, and was decked with flowers, violets in particular, which were supposed to have sprung from the blood of Attis. On the third day, the 24th March, came the 'Day of Blood', when the high priest drew blood from his arm and presented it as an offering. The clergy joined in, with clashing cymbals, flutes, drums and horns, and whirled around in a dance, slashing themselves with knives. The offering of blood was meant to bring Attis back to life, or at least hasten his journey towards resurrection in the next life. This story is further substantiated by the legend that Attis was conceived when Cybele placed a pomegranate in her bosom, grown from the severed genitals of Agdistis, a man-monster. This practice led to many other instances of Asiatic goddesses of fertility being served by eunuch priests.

During an archaeological dig of two mounds in Turkey in 1957, author and historian James Mellaart discovered the ancient ruins of Çatal Hüyük. This was a highly organised and sophisticated Stone Age city in the Anatolian Highlands of Central Turkey 575 BCE, described by Mellaart as, 'like a supernova among the rather dim galaxy of peasant cultures,' (*Earliest Civilisations of The East*, James Mellaart, 1965). It was here that archaeologists found one of the earliest representations of a fertility image, a terracotta figure of the goddess Cybele seated on a throne, represented as the mistress of both wild and domestic animals. Her breasts, hips and belly are voluminous, and from between her massive legs she appears to be giving birth while resting her hands on the heads of leopards on either side of her. Cybele was also associated with hunting, fertility and the moon, and priestesses worshipped her on each lunar cycle honouring the monthly cycle of women. Cybele became the Romans' supreme patron, and the cult of the great fertility god and mother of gods from Phrygia in Asia Minor could be traced back to early neolithic times. The wild orgiastic ceremonies of her followers shocked the Roman senate with their frenzied dances. These were accompanied by rattles, drums and tambourines, as well as howling and screeching.

According to James Mellaart and his team of archaeologists who discovered Çatal Hüyük, it was impossible to establish where the extremely organised, sophisticated and highly skilled Stone Age craftsmen and farmers came from. The numerous figurines and other artefacts excavated from the site were evidence of an ancient civilisation with an elaborate religion that focused on the dual aspect of the mother goddess who manifested herself as both maiden and mother, as both the source of life and its manifestation.

The Cult of the Phallus

In Greece, the cult of the phallus belonged mainly to the god Dionysus. This included many elements of fantasy, tragedy and comedy that probably sprang from early idolisation and worship of female genitalia and reproductive powers. On a Greek vase painting, a woman is depicted dancing before an enthroned Dionysus wearing an artificial phallus. Another painting depicts a nude woman striding out carrying a very large phallus under her arm. The Dionysiac religion successfully thrived to become the most popular pagan ritual of the Graeco-Roman world (*The Reign of the Phallus, Sexual Politics of Ancient Athens*, Eva C. Keuls, 1993). Evidence of the type of dances mentioned earlier, where dancers attach a bast phallus to simulate the sex act, has been found in the Villa of the Mysteries, outside Pompeii on the Seventh Panel, showing scenes such as 'The Phallus Unveiled' and 'The Lifting of the Rod', discovered in 1930. Phallic dances were extremely erotic; in some phallic rites, sexual intercourse took place.

Phallic dances had their roots in religion. They were a symbol of fertility, a means of celebrating life forces in the belief that they would stimulate fertility, ward off evil and protect the dancers against disease and the destruction of their communities. Such dances persisted for thousands of years but unfortunately are now almost extinct. Much of their decline can be attributed to Christian missionaries who over the centuries outlawed such tribal dances as heathen debaucheries. To these ancient people, however, the dances were not obscene or sensational pleasures but matters of life and unity with the great mother earth on whom they depended for their survival.

Numerous gods and goddesses of Ancient Greece found their way to Rome. Among them was Artemis, who became Diana, symbolising strength of character, Aphrodite, who became Venus, the goddess of love and womanhood, and Hera who transformed into Juno, the goddess of marriage and childbirth.

Psychological and Physical Aspects of Dance

The psychological and physical side of dance is often over-looked but for centuries dance was accepted as a cure for many conditions. In the Middle Ages, outbreaks of famine and plague were frequent, affecting thousands of people. When the condition abated, the population, which had been overwrought with anxiety bordering on mass hysteria, took to the streets where they began to dance with little restraint. Mania would take over as they danced themselves into a delirious state until collapsing with sheer exhaustion. These ecstatic and manic dances continued well into the late Middle Ages until they were banned because they were considered to be depraved.

'The Tarantella' from Southern Italy was a dance that became popular among young girls in Germany and Italy between the 15th and 17th century. They used tambourines and castanets to accompany the dance. It is thought to have originated from the movements of those suffering convulsions from the venomous bite of the tarantula spider, which took its name from the city of Tarantella. *The Standard Oxford English Dictionary* defines the term as follows: 'Tarantism (1638)… A hysterical malady, characterized by an extreme impulse to dance, which prevailed as an epidemic in Apulia and adjacent parts of Italy from the 15th to the 17th century, popularly attributed to the bite or 'sting' of the tarantula'.

Those who were bitten by the spider suffered terrible pain resulting in convulsive twitching, jerking and jumping around. To help victims deal with the excruciating pain and prevent them from going insane, musicians were immediately summoned to play for them while they impulsively danced, as it was believed their music would help them through their painful ordeal. The locals frequently joined in the dancing to help release their tensions and frustrations until overcome by exhaustion.

The uncontrollable shaking and trembling of Saint Vitus' disease (erroneously named after Saint Vitus whose saint's day happened to coincide with Saint John's day or Midsummer's Day) was characterised by irregular involuntary contractions of the muscles. It is properly known as chorea, which the

Oxford Concise Medical Dictionary defines as follows: 'A jerky involuntary movement, particularly affecting the shoulders, hips and face. Each movement is sudden but the resulting posture may be prolonged for a few seconds. The symptoms are due to disease of the basal ganglia.' This convulsive disorder of the Middle Ages was also described as a 'dance of hysterics' which spread to such epidemic proportions that the clergy and physicians were unable to help.

The story of the Pied Piper from Hamlyn is based on a legend relating to dance mania. After dancing to exhaustion, the sufferers fell into a deep sleep that relieved them of their symptoms. In an endeavour to bring this disorder to a climax as soon as possible, the services of musicians were hired to play for those inflicted by the malady until they dropped.

Many religious experiences were physical and expressed mainly through dance which then became a sacrificial rite.

Conclusion

For people of the ancient civilisations, the greatest goddess of all was the earth mother, the mother of the universe, on whom they relied for their survival. They believed she was the creator of all things, the rebirth of humanity and nature and the controller of life's force and death. The cult of the mother goddess survived for thousands of years and she was fervently worshipped in the form of dance, song and music. It was universally believed that without her sustaining power life could not have existed in any form.

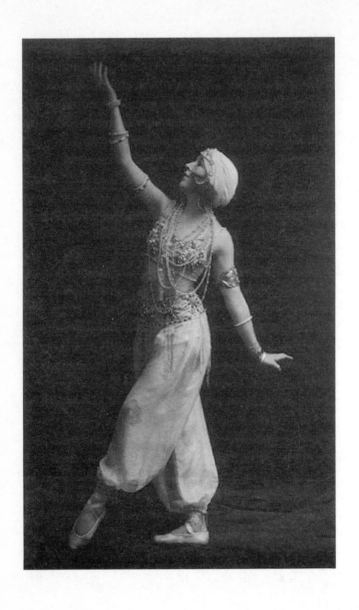

2

The Sacred Dance

Various forms of the belly dance, which grew out of ancient rituals and folk dances over the centuries, have remained an important part of culture and tradition throughout Middle Eastern communities. These days the belly dance is performed primarily for entertainment purposes, often as a commercial venture in cabaret form in nightclubs, restaurants, weddings and other celebrations.

In Ancient Egypt, dance was an expression of joy and an integral part of magic, religious rituals and funeral rites. Egyptians loved pomp and ceremony and in every town and village troupes of male and female dancers, conjurors, gymnasts and acrobats were employed to perform during elaborate religious processions and festivities. There are numerous illustrations on tomb walls and monument reliefs which attest to the dancers' great physical strength, skill, agility and energy.

During royal processions in honour of the gods it was everyone's duty to dance and so the king himself would participate, on occasion contributing a 'Dance of the Gods.' A relief from the Narmer Pallette 3000 BCE, for example, depicts the king apparently taking part in a procession of standard-bearers (*British Museum Dictionary of Ancient Egypt*, Ian Shaw and Paul Nicholson,1995) and a relief of the 18th

Dynasty (1550–1295 BCE) shows King Tuthmosis IV dancing before the goddess Hathor.

Included amongst the professions from which Ancient Egyptian women were able to choose were the roles of priestess, which gained the highest honour, professional mourner, midwife, musician or dancer. If the women chose dancing as a profession, whether on an amateur or professional basis, they were respected and highly regarded.

One of the most famous Egyptian dance scenes known, as depicted in the tomb of Nenkhehtifkai at Saqqara, is that of four female dancers accompanied by female musicians performing at a banquet. The dancers are positioned one behind the other, each standing on one leg with the other elevated high in front, and inclining backwards with arms outstretched in a position parallel to the elevated leg. Their long, dark, plaited hair is tied with a weighted disc and swings behind them, emphasising the degree of their arched backs. This type of Egyptian dance with discs is depicted on a Middle Kingdom relief from the tomb of Queen Neferu of the 18th Dynasty, which shows performers with a string of ornaments in their hair, which were, according to the historian Cyril Aldred, large silver discs (*Jewels of the Pharoahs*, Cyril Aldred, 1971). What we cannot deduce is whether the dancers are preparing to take a long stride or are intending to execute a backbend, cartwheel or somersault.

When performing, the dancers' routines would often include amazing acrobatics. In reliefs from temples of the Pharaonic Period for example, dancers are pictured doing handstands, cartwheels, somersaults and back flips and back bends (bellydancemusem.com). Other movements such as arching backwards, forwards and sideways and swinging the upper torso to and fro whilst keeping the back rigid could be altered to include slow, circular movements of the hips and upper torso. Acrobatic dancing was extremely popular in the

New Kingdom (1550–1069 BCE) together with an erotic style of dancing also featured on reliefs from this period showing young women wearing nothing more than sheer, transparent ankle-length dresses and playing tambourines and castanets as they danced. Their sensuous, snake-like movements appear to have been similar to those performed by oriental dancers today.

There is evidence from reliefs of this period of girls in their very early childhood dancing, sometimes naked, as they entertain company. The lower register of the 6th Dynasty relief from the tomb of Mastaba of Mereroku, one of the largest tombs at the Saqqara site, shows five very young girls doing Hathor dances, holding hand-shaped wooden rattles in their left hands and mirrors in their right hands. Evidence of the fondness of the very young for dancing is also provided in the masterly carving at the bottom of an oblong wooden box of unknown function found at Saqqara also and attributed on stylistic grounds to the 18th Dynasty (*Egyptian State Information Service*, 2003).

Amongst adults also, nude dancing was fairly common in Ancient Egypt. Most Egyptians of the time were neither shocked nor intimidated by the nudity of others. In the New Kingdom (1550–1069 BCE) it was not unusual for women of a low status employed in well-to-do households to be naked or semi-naked as they went about their daily business. Women of higher rank were also uninhibited about appearing semi-clad in public as seen in the 12th Dynasty relief showing Princess Sebeknakht breast-feeding her child and in the unique Armana relief featuring Queen Nefertiti feeding one of her six daughters around 1350 BCE (The Regents of the University of California, www.ucop.edu, 2003).

The bridge, a popular movement performed by Ancient Egyptian dancers, involved a backbend from a standing position. As the dancer or acrobat arched backwards, he or she would swing the arms up and over their head until the hands reached the floor. While in this position, the dancers would walk on all fours in any direction, propelling themselves by using their hands and feet, then pulling themselves up to a vertical position. This kind of acrobatic feat is referred to by historians such as J. Gardner Wilkinson in his report of 1837 and by Eugen Strouhal in *The Lives of the Ancient Egyptians* (1992), who describes the moves of dancers as 'elegant, graceful, even acrobatic.'

The cradle is another well-illustrated Ancient Egyptian dance movement, which the dancer would execute by lying on the floor and swinging both legs up together until they touched the back of the head. Then, having grabbed both ankles firmly, the dancer was able to rock to and fro on the belly. Both the bridge and cradle moments are still performed by gymnasts and acrobats today. They are extremely strenuous and should only be attempted if you are very fit and supple.

Pyramid formation was, and still is, included in the highly gymnastic dances of the Gnawa, which have magical and religious connotations. The Gnawa are inhabitants of Morocco who are mainly descendents of dark-skinned Negroid slaves brought from the South. The Gnawa are organised as a religious fraternity and according to a written account by anthropologist Eugene Aubins, they are skilled in medicine and also include fortune-tellers and exorcists who cast out demons and evil spirits. Infertile women often consult a female prophet or 'fatika' who is believed able to predict the future. Sensational gymnastic feats continue to be performed in public by the Gnawa during festivals. The dancers, men and young boys, seek to outperform each other with their physical feats that demand energy, dexterity, precision and balance. Dancers climb up on the heads and shoulders of their companions until a great height is reached and they attain the shape of the pyramid. Once they have achieved their goal, they descend by jumping down one after the other in quick succession, immediately tumbling into cartwheels, somersaults and back-flips. The performance is concluded by solo exhibitions of their acrobatic skills.

Towards the end of the 4th century BCE a young man from Syracuse, whose name is not known, was invited to a banquet in Memphis by a rich Egyptian. There he observed such a display and wrote the following account of it, as translated by Irena Lexova from the German version by Fritz Wegge:

'Suddenly they disappeared and in their place came forward a group of dancers who jumped about in all directions, gathered together again, climbed one of top of the other with an incredible dexterity, mounting on the shoulders and the heads, forming pyramids reaching to the ceiling of the hall, then descending one after the other to perform new jumps and [other moves called] 'saltomortales'. Being in constant motion, now they danced on their hands, now they gathered in pairs, one turning his head down between the legs of his mate, then they lifted themselves mutually and reclined to the original position, each of them alternately being lifted and upon falling lifting his partner up.' (*Ancient Egyptian Dances*, Irena Lexova, 1975).

Henry Wild, a Swiss Egyptologist who studied the dances of the Pharaonic Period (*Les Danses Sacres de L'Egypt Ancienne*, Henry Wild, 1963 and *Women in Ancient Egypt*, Barbara Watterson, 1998) concluded that these ancient dances consisted of hops, leaps, strides, jumps, pirouettes and slow, circular movements of the trunk that were done while the feet remained still. He also noted that while walking on the balls of their feet, the dancers' arms were raised in a curved position above their heads – the same arm movement that Oriental dancers use today. He believed that these dances were part of a sequence executed methodically, step by step, when dancing in groups or pairs.

On a relief of the 5th Dynasty (2494-2345 BCE) from Saqqara a group of girls are shown dancing in pairs facing one another and holding hands as they support themselves on one leg. Their other leg is lifted up in front of them, bent at the knee, with their toes touching their partner. It is not clear what movement they made next.

A dance known only as the IB3 (*Music and Musicians in Ancient Egypt*, Lise Manniche, 1991) involves two typical steps performed by dancers of the Pharaonic Period. It is depicted on a relief that shows a dancer whose foot is slightly lifted up from the floor with both arms raised above her head. Another dancer has her leg lifted much higher and is holding her arms in the same position as her partner. Although it was more common to have both arms raised when dancing, dancers are sometimes seen with just one arm lifted. Pre-dynastic (4000-3100 BCE) vessels and clay figurines also portray dancing females with arms raised above their heads. Male dancers such as the Khawals (who are female impersonators from Egypt) and the Ginks (who are also female impersonators, though not of Egyptian blood), have always danced in a similar way to female dancers, moving towards one another until they stood directly opposite each other on one leg. It is likely they stamped the foot, stood on the other leg, and then repeated the step before proceeding with a series of other movements.

Whether in pairs or in groups of four or more, dancers were also pictured with clenched fists and touching each other only with their thumbs. The dancers may have changed partners at some point during their dance; what is difficult to ascertain is whether each dancer's movements were independent of their partners. Scenes that have survived from Ancient Egypt almost never portray members of both sexes dancing together; they always appear to dance separately.

In group dancing we find dancers playing musical instruments such as the lute, double reed pipes or wooden clappers, which would doubtless have restricted their freedom of movement. In some dances associated with the goddess Hathor a mirror was held in one hand, used to reflect the other hand or another object held in the other hand.

Some dances of the Middle Kingdom (2055–1650 BCE), illustrated on tombs at Beni Hasan, show women juggling balls. Balls were also used in the Old Kingdom (2686–2160 BCE) and were shown to be attached to the dancers' long, plaited hair, which they swung from side to side and brushed along the ground as they rotated their upper torsos around in large sweeping circles.

Egyptians performed lyrical dances at banquets. A description of one such dance is given from the letter written by the young man from Syracuse and as translated from the German version by Fritz Wegge:

'Now I caught sight of a troupe of musicians, coming with various instruments in their hands, in which I recognised harps, guitars, lyres, simple and double pipes, tambourines and cymbals. We were overwhelmed constantly by songs which were most cordially applauded by the audience. Then, at a given sign, the middle of the hall was taken by a man and girl dancer, who were provided with clappers. These were made out of two small pieces of wood, round and concave, located in the palms and giving rhythm to the dancing when suddenly knocked together. These two dancers danced separately or together in harmonious configurations, mixed with pirouettes, soon parting and again approaching one another, the young dancer turning and running after his mate and following her with expressions of tender desire, while she fled from him constantly, rotating and pirouetting, as if refusing his endeavours after amorous approach. This performance was done lightly and energetically in harmonious postures, and seemed to me exceedingly entertaining.' (*Ancient Egyptian Dances*, Irena Lexova, 1975.)

Dances in Ancient Egypt played an essential role in funeral rituals, which are thought to date from pre-dynastic times. Such dances were based on the belief that life continued beyond death and were representative of the energy of the sun, which was a symbol of life. In the Old Kingdom (2686-2160 BCE), these dances were performed by a number of male and female professional dancers who were hired especially for such occasions. During the funeral procession they would perform graceful, sensuous and wild acrobatic movements, accompanied by others with rhythmic clapping, chanting, the shaking of rattles and waving of olive branches.

Funeral dances were performed to celebrate rebirth and the renewal of life and to entertain and honour the dead. They played a vital role in expressing the grief of the mourners. During the funeral rituals the bereaved were supported by very young girls hired as professional mourners who congregated to grieve openly in the homes of the dead. They also stood among the mourners with arms raised above their heads, swaying from side to side while wailing and chanting as loud as their lungs would permit. The Ka was an individual's vital force that accompanied him or her in both life and death (*The Art and Architecture of Ancient Egypt*, W. Stevenson Smith, 1981). The dances of the Ka took place at funerals. The dancers would interlink arms and perform a chain dance around the funeral pyre. The ritual movements, as in other funeral dances, followed in the direction of the sun's course, symbolising the unity of life and death.

Some reliefs depict the king and gods as participants in the dancing and festivities. For example, in reliefs from the temple of Luxor depicting Opet festivities of the Theban area (which are recorded as taking place from the start of the New Kingdom onwards) dances of the king during the 18th Dynasty are documented. Here he is pictured performing a 'Dance of the Gods,' before the god Amun-Re of Karnak and is shown kneeling to receive various crowns from the god and making special offerings in return, a ritual performed as a means of reasserting the ties between deity and royalty (*Complete Temples of Ancient Egypt*, Richard H. Wilkinson, 2000). Amongst the gods who have joined in the festivities is Bes, the dwarf god, whose grotesque and hideous appearance amused everyone and whose noisy tambourine shaking was said to frighten away demons. 'Bes was a genial bearded creature partly human in form, but with the tail, mane and ears of a lion,' (*The Art and Architecture of Ancient Egypt*, W. Stevenson Smith, 1981).

Evidence collated from depictions of funerals suggests that the origin of these sacred dances originated from pre-dynastic times. One in particular known as the Muu dance was performed by men only, often wearing tall, green head-dresses made from reeds and short, pointed skirts or kilts as seen in a detail from the New Kingdom scene at the Tomb of Tetiki (*The Dance in Ancient Egypt*, Emma Brenner-Traut, 1938). Professional dancer and dance scholar Elizabeth 'Artemis' Mornat categorized the dances of Ancient Egypt into six types: religious, non-religious festival, banquet, harem, combat and street dances, claiming the Muu dancers were a vital part of funerary processions (www.showcase.netins.net 2003).

A painting from the tombs of Saqqara (2500 BCE) now held in the museum of Cairo, shows two young girls leading a funeral procession. Whilst holding rattles they are surrounded by a circle of women wearing transparent dresses and holding tambourines in their hands as they perform ecstatic and sensual dance movements.

The striding dance was also performed at funerals, its

function being to ensure the sun's uninterrupted course across the sky. This dance was also performed by the pharaohs, who solemnly danced with long strides around the walls of their temple during the funeral rituals. Women also danced, taking long strides and raising their legs high above their heads as they accompanied a coffin in the hope of winning eternal life for the dead.

In his book, *Life of the Ancient Egyptians* (1992), Eugen Strouhal describes the mourning ceremonies of the Fellahin of Upper Egypt, direct descendants of the temple builders of Ancient Thebes (*Shakhat: An Egyptian*, Richard Critchfield, 1990) and whom he had the privilege of witnessing on several occasions. He wrote that during the period of mourning, which lasted several days, the female mourners gathered together in the home of the deceased or in a secluded spot outdoors where they would wail, utter piercing cries and dance. They would sway forwards and backwards, moving around in a circle whilst striking their faces with both hands to the accompaniment of hysterical cries and chants. Sometimes one of the dancers would beat out a rhythm on a single membrane drum that resembled a tambourine without its jingles.

In the Pharaonic Period, the styles of dance depicted in painting and carvings presented only two-thirds or three-quarters of their profile, rendering the appearance of the dancers and their movements expressionless and angular. This was because all the scenes were portrayed as active, such as praying, dancing, labouring, talking with another figure or making offerings to the gods. By working in profile, artists avoided a three-dimensional aspect that they believed should be only for portraits of the gods. To these Ancient Egyptian artists it was important that they sustained the traditions of their ancestors. New ideas that diverged from the norm were unacceptable, especially in art.

Dance in Ancient Egypt was both sophisticated and varied. Apart from the Egyptians' own ritual, magical and sacred dances, and those of the pygmies that were brought into Egypt, a new dance emerged, introduced by the 'Bayaderes' or Hindu temple dancers, who were young girls brought by the Egyptians from the conquered regions of the East to Egypt around 1500 BCE. Their style of dance had none of the long measures, strides or rhomboid movements as depicted on numerous Egyptian stone reliefs including those on the picture of dancers from the Tomb of Kagemni at Saqqara. Their movements, not dissimilar to those performed today by dancers worldwide, were far more undulating, snake-like and graceful, thus introducing a much softer, more feminine style of dance to Egypt.

Influences from Around the World

In Luxor in the Theban area of Upper Egypt my students and I had a unique opportunity to join a group of male dancers celebrating a local wedding. We danced behind one another in a long line, with each of our right hands resting on the shoulder of the person in front, doing a tiny step I have seen in other tribal dances that I can only describe as akin to limping. Keeping the right foot flat and the heel of the left foot raised, we pushed out our left hips as we transferred the weight from right to left. The movement was very repetitive and the dance seemed to last for hours but although we were all exhausted and ended up with aching right legs, we enjoyed it immensely.

I was also unexpectedly invited by the well-known group 'Musicians of the Nile' and local professional dancers to dance on this special occasion, a great honour and privilege. I was touched by the response I received from the locals and musicians after my performance. It was an occasion I shall never forget. During the same week, a group of us had the opportunity to take part in a Nubian and Aswanic folklore dance workshop run by a group of male dancers. Having the opportunity to learn some ancient Nubian dances was great fun and a wonderful experience.

Nubia was the most southern part of Egypt and, as early as the 1st Dynasty (3000-2890 BCE), had always been of great interest to the Egyptians. Trade routes and the demand for raw materials such as ivory, ebony, perfumes, incense and gold (the Nubians' most valuable asset) were a source of contention between the southern people and the pharaohs. In the Middle Kingdom (2055-1650 BCE) the Egyptians conquered Nubia and the area became an Egyptian province. In time, the Nubians, who were mainly employed as slaves and miners, adopted the manners and customs of the Egyptians. Around 730 BCE the Nubians tired of being under the influence of the pharaohs and took control of much of Egypt. Approximately seventy years later, the Assyrians ended the supremacy of the Nubians who returned to their own country and eventually reverted back to their own culture.

The Nubians brought with them their own tribal dances. Their dance steps were regulated by rhythmic hand clapping and drum beats. The cane dance performed by male Nubian dancers is energetic and involves leaps, turns, and kicks, as well as their twirling the cane as they lie on the floor, arching into a backbend from a kneeling position. In contrast, the Nubian female cane dance is a little more genteel, with jump steps, alternate kicks, hip pushes and shimmies. The cane is held at either end and the dancer raises it above her head or places it out in front of herself.

For centuries, a traditional cane dance called Raqs as Assaya originating in Saida, Upper Egypt, during the Pharaonic Period, has been performed by Islamic, African and Asian female dancers. This dance is an acrobatic version of the cane dance and in recent years it has become increasingly popular with male and female dancers in the West. It is promoted across the globe by traditional Egyptian dancers such as the popular male dancer Sayed el Joker, for example, now a resident of Germany. The cane used is usually a standard wooden walking stick with a crook end that is about three feet (one metre) in length and is sometimes elaborately decorated for effect with sequins, brightly coloured ribbon or tape. Whilst dancing, the female dancer balances the cane on her head, holds it above her body and across her shoulders as she travels forwards or backwards. If the dancer is very co-ordinated, she masterfully twirls the cane around as she shimmies or rapidly moves her hips. Some dancers are known to balance the cane across their breasts or abdomen as they ripple and roll it, making for pure cabaret. This style of cane dancing has no symbolic significance but highlights the co-ordination and dexterity of the female dancer. Solo male dancers also perform a stick dance similar to that of the females, using the cane to complement and show off their movements. The dance involves robust action of the pelvic area, thrusting backwards, forwards, up and down.

The Egyptian male stick dance Raks Tahtib is highly symbolic, representing combat, and is performed by two dancers at one time and originally using swords. Nowadays, a stick or pole of up to five feet in length is used to represent a weapon wielded during hunting or for battle, where the two male opponents take part in a mock fight. Raks Tahtib requires much concentration, agility and skill and is a variant of the Tahtib, a highly competitive and theatrical dance which tourists rarely have the opportunity to observe. It is played as a serious 'game' in which participants are not obliged to abide by all the rules. While the dancers prepare for the show, the leader of the Mizmar band (rayyis), plays a short solo introduction that sets up the melody and tempo, eventually leading into the Egyptian national anthem. When the dancers are ready to begin the whole ensemble plays. Each musician intently watches every move the dancers make so they can adapt their rhythm to the pace of the fighters. As the dance begins, each dancer takes a stick, held in either one or both hands. The dancers then begin to swing and wave it above their heads as they move around in circles. This initial part of the dance is their way of greeting one another. The dancers then proceed with the 'battle' in earnest, varying their movements as they swiftly whirl around, jumping energetically and falling down onto their knees in an effort to dodge their opponents and to avoid being struck. As they twirl their sticks in circles around them, they strive to strike a blow on any part of their opponents' bodies, an action called 'kasf'.

To help protect themselves from being struck, the dancers are allowed to slide one hand down the lower end of the stick. This enables them to hold it in a horizontal position with both hands. Whenever one of the dancers succeeds in hitting an opponent he scores a point and if either of them touches the side or back of an opponent they are awarded extra points. When a dancer is struck by an opponent's stick he has to make a concerted effort to strike his opponent back to even the score. If the dancer succeeds he wins a point, and the result is a match draw (known as a 'gita') but if he fails to draw he loses the game. It has been known for dancers to collapse through sheer exhaustion during this strenuous, extremely energetic dance.

There are various combative dances, one of which involves two men taking part in a mock duel over a woman. As they fight, the flirtatious female responsible for the duel dances in and around the men, provoking them even further.

Many theories have emerged as to the origins of the next combatative dance we shall discuss, which is called 'The Sword

Dance'. Linked sword dances are believed to have developed in Europe, whereas it is thought that mock battle dances originated in the Middle East, Japan and North Africa centuries ago. Varieties of sword dance still performed today include the Baccu Ber dance from the French Alps, with its forty-five figures, the Bagnasco dance from Italy and various others from the Czech Republic and Slovakia. Many versions of ritual Morris Dance and other sword dances have survived in England until the present day.

Sword dances were first danced by men and there is little information available to ascertain when or why women first performed the dance. One possible explanation is that the Bedouins of Eastern Sudan, skilled metal workers who excelled in producing fine swords, demonstrated their craftsmanship to potential buyers by balancing swords on their daughters' heads; a custom which is though to have developed into a symbolic dance of swords. Alternatively, it may have been that this dance was performed by daughters in honour of their fathers' prowess as warriors or craftsmen. As the girl danced, she would skilfully balance the sharp-edged sword upon her head and carry another one in her hand, as depicted in an exquisite painting, *La Dance du Sabre* (1895), by Jean-Leon Gerome, a traveller and oriental artist (1824–1904). In his book, *Rashaayda Bedouin: Arab Pastoralists of Eastern Sudan*, (1995), William Charles Young describes a sword dance of both men and women as a ritualistic dance used to impress members of the opposite sex.

In the Middle East, swords were part of upper class dress for men as well as weapons used in combat. On occasion, male dancers, who were usually poor people from the lower classes, were hired to entertain the soldiers. As the nights drew in and the soldiers became inebriated, they would lend their sharp-edged swords to the dancers who balanced them upon their heads – and more often than not sneaked off into the night with them. It is claimed, by dance experts such as Caroline Varga Dinicu, also known as 'Morocco' and author of numerous publications on dance, that dancers stockpiled these swords for real combat against their upper class oppressors but that after a couple of uprisings, the local Pasha, a high official of the Ottoman Empire, announced that anyone seen dancing with a sword on his head would have his head chopped off. It was feared by the officials that the cache of swords would be used in an uprising against them, hence the disappearance of sword dances in the Middle East and North Africa for a while.

Another type of sword dance called 'The Weapon Dance' was a religious rite that was practised in many early civilisations and required much skill and agility. These dances were divided into non-mimetic and circling dances as in the following example of a weapon dance of the Khasi of Upper Burma who moved very slowly in a circle. At intervals the dancers would shout, then separate into pairs, leaping towards one another and striking their swords before yelling loudly, moving back and continuing to circle.

Written evidence of this type of ritual ceremonial dancing came from Roman and Greek writers, who describe the priestly dancing of the Korbantes, Daktyles on Mount Ida and the Kuretes of the Dictean Caves. These rituals were a means of expelling winter and its accompanying evils and inviting in spring by noisily clashing their swords against their shields (*Discovering English Folk Dance*, Hugh Rippon Shire, 1975).

There are still some Saudi dancers who have preserved the traditional sword dance. One in particular was an elderly man whom the famous Egyptian dancer, Magna Sala, featured in her film on belly dance. While holding the sword in his hands and tensing his muscles, the man could make the sword shimmer until it appeared irradiated, which must have been incredible to watch.

H.V. Morton (1892-1979), a traveller and writer, witnessed a strange and dangerous type of knife dance, performed at a wedding celebration in a village called Zosta during his visit to Turkey in 1936 (*In the Steps of St Paul*, H.V. Morton, 1936). Morton described the dancer as a young man dressed in a woman's red silk dress, with his face heavily rouged and eyes blackened with kohl. He looked as fierce as a wild cat. To the monotonous but hypnotic beat of a drum, he flashed and clashed his knives together aggressively, shaking his body and stamping his feet as he whirled and twirled around the room in a frenzied manner. He then pretended to stab a member of the audience, which Morton described as a savage sight. Suddenly, he leapt and crouched before another member of the audience, waving his knives treacherously close to his eyes and throat.

In Algeria, a 'Dance of Fighters' is performed with sabres and rifles by the Oulad horsemen, dressed in traditional costume and armed with rifles. They gallop at great speed around an arena, performing spectacular acrobatic feats that leave one breathless. As the show reaches its climax, the horsemen thunder down the length of the arena, stopping suddenly within yards of the spectators to fire their rifles into the air. You literally jump out of your seat. Unfortunately, over the centuries, the history and original meaning of this ancient Berber ritual has been lost. A similar dance is that of the Ghiatas warriors of Morocco who dance with guns in their hands to drums and mussettes (a smaller, French version of the bagpipes), yelling rhythmic but muffled sounds. The dance, like many other warrior dances, comes to a climax with a volley of gunfire.

The Sacred Flame

For thousands of years, torches and candles were used during ceremonial, religious and secular rituals around the world.

They are still used in many religious ceremonies today. The flames of torches and candles were believed by ancient people to be symbolic of the divine and energising power of the sun, and represent light and warmth.

In Ancient Greece, the Maenads (madwomen), female members of the orgiastic cult of Dionysus, carried flaming torches during their frenzied ritual dances.

In Turkey during a bride's 'henna' preparation for her nuptials, her family and friends perform a circle dance during which they hold lighted candles. As in many other Middle Eastern cultures, henna decoration and lighted candles are believed to ward off evil.

In the Middle East, North Africa and Persia, dances still exist in which candles are reverently used. One such traditional dance is the Moroccan 'Tea Tray Dance', a symbolic ceremony of making and pouring tea. In the centre of a large tray embellished with sprigs of mint leaves, a tall silver or brass teapot stands with several glass cups around it containing mint tea or lighted candles. While balancing the tray upon his or her head, the dancer undulates, thrusts the hips and shimmies provocatively. When I witnessed this on a recent visit to Morocco, I was amazed by the skill of one particular dancer. As I watched her she went down on her knees arching back into a backbend and shimmied her body from tip to toe, all the while balancing the tray on her head. This particular dance is performed by either men or women and I have seen it in Turkey, Morocco and New York.

Another dance in which candles are used spectacularly is the Raks al Shemadan, more commonly known as 'The Candelabrum Dance'. This requires skill, balance and strength, particularly of the neck and spine, to enable the dancer to perform it confidently. The authentic candelabrum is a heavy branched ornamental candlestick, approximately three feet (one metre) high, made from brass or other metals.

Embellished with at least twelve tall, illuminated candles, the candelabrum sits firmly on the head of the dancer as she shimmies her hips and shoulders and undulates to the rhythm of the music.

Although this dance is believed to have originated from France about one hundred years ago, it is also said to have been performed in Turkey under Ottoman rule. The dance is very popular with Egyptian artists. It was a favourite of the star performer Shaffi al Ibtiyya, a wealthy but infamous Egyptian dancer of the 1920s who worked as a belly dancer in Egypt's first official nightclub, the 'Eldorado'. In her performances of the Raks al Shemadan she was able to do the splits while balancing the candelabrum on her head. Sadly, she died in poverty in 1962.

Morocco, Land of Contrasts

Belly dancing as performed today throughout Morocco is likely to have evolved from the various Berber folk dances as it did in the Middle East and also from other cultural influences established over the course of the country's history by invaders such as the Phoenicians and the Spaniards. Morocco, the 'Gateway to Africa', is a beautiful, fascinating and enticing country, comprising many different civilisations and complex cultures that go back over 3000 years. Bordered by both the Atlantic and the Mediterranean, it is located at the North Western tip of Africa. The Atlas Mountains form the backbone of Morocco. The highest peaks tower over 11,500 feet (3500 metres) and cover a distance of 450 miles (700 kilometres). These magnificent mountains with their deep gorges, high peaks and valleys, define the border between the southern half of the country, with its expanse of hot, inhospitable desert, and the mild oceanic climate of the fertile northern part of the country, with its green pastures and small lakes, where fragrant pine, eucalyptus, olive and palm trees flourish.

Winter in the mountains becomes very harsh and formidable, as the snow falls heavily on the high plains of the Atlas. In late spring as the temperature rises, the thaw produces spectacular waterfalls that cascade into the ravines, creating flowing rivers that become a natural source for reservoirs and which generate enough power to supply most of Morocco. Three out of the four mountain ranges, High Atlas, Middle Atlas and the Rif give rise to magnificent forests of the evergreen oak, holm, and also cedar, to create spectacular scenery. The impressive crescent-shaped Rif mountain range separates Northern Morocco from the rest of the country and rises directly behind Fes and Meknes. Riffian or Riffi people, who speak Riff or Senhaja, inhabit the Rif Mountains.

Throughout its history, Morocco has had many upheavals. From the 6th century BCE onwards, the country has been occupied by many different races, though the earliest recorded inhabitants are the North African Berber tribe. In 1100 BCE, they were subjugated by the Phoenician immigrants who settled in Morocco, calling them 'Mahurin' meaning 'Westerners' and setting up trading posts along the coastline. These Phoenician settlements, which eventually became part of the Carthaginian Empire, were conquered by the Romans in 146 BCE, so that Roman rule prevailed until the fall of the Roman Empire in the 5th century. (The Romans named the Berbers 'Numidea'.) In 670 CE, Oqba Ben Nafi and his Muslim armies arrived, eventually establishing a Muslim Empire. A century later, Idris Ben Abdallah, supposedly a descendent of the prophet Mohammed Ali's son-in-law, became the first sultan of the Islamic kingdom of Maghreb el-Aqsa - Arabic for 'The Extreme West'. He helped spread the word of Islam, which has remained dominant throughout Moroccan culture since.

By 1060 CE, Yusuf Ibn Tashfin, a Moroccan leader from the dynasty of the Almoravids, united the whole country and declared Marrakech the capital of Morocco. He set out to conquer lands as far down as Algiers and eventually West Africa and Spain, capturing Argel before invading Andalusia in 1086 CE. During the early 16th century, the Spanish and Portuguese controlled Morocco's ports. In the 18th century, Moulay Ismail governed the country. He was a man with great vision who established diplomatic links with Europe and other countries. One hundred years later in 1912, Spain controlled part of Northern Morocco, while the rest of the country was colonised by the French until 1956. After an unsettled period, the country became independent in 1956. In 1961 Hassan II, again believed to be a descendant of the great prophet Ali, became king and religious leader of Morocco.

In a country that has been subject to countless invasions and influences over the course of its history, the Berbers have successfully maintained their own dialects, traditions and unique way of life. 'Berber' is a general name used for different people throughout North Africa, including the Taureg Nomads and peasants of Kabylie in Algeria. Originating from East Africa and the Orient, the Moroccan Berbers are direct descendants from the Sahnhadja, Masmuda and Zanuta, Nafza, Hawwara and Luwata tribes and are split into many tribes often called Beni or 'sons of'.

For many centuries, generations of Berbers have handed down their rich folklore of wisdom and poetry to their people. They live in close harmony with nature. Using traditional farming methods, they prepare the land for crops of maize, wheat, barley and vegetables by ploughing their fields as their ancestors did long ago. From July to September, when the harvest has been reaped and work in the fields has finished, festivals and celebrations take place in towns and remote villages the length and breadth of the Atlas Mountains.

One of the most famous events is the Moussem, also known as the 'Fair of Fiancées', held in the town of Imilchil in the High Atlas, the administrative centre of the Ait Hadiddou tribe. This is a lively festival lasting for several days that attracts thousands of people looking for an opportunity to find a marriage partner, as well as giving each Berber tribe the chance to show their agricultural crafts and produce. Marriage plays a very important role in Berber society. By uniting a couple in marriage, the stability of the Berber community is guaranteed for future generations. The streets and market squares bustle with traders selling their crafts, fabrics, cattle and grains, along with fortune tellers, entertainers and men parading their charms in the hope of attracting a beautiful woman. For hours on end, groups of musicians beat out pulsating rhythms on goblet-shaped percussion instruments and frame drums, held in one hand and struck by the other. Wind instruments such as the flute are played to accompany singers, who recite poetic songs. In contrast to the singers, the dancers sway to a slower tempo, called the Ahouach, one of the main forms of music and dance (along with the Ahaidous) performed in the High Atlas. It hails from the Great Atlas Valley and is also known as the 'shadow dance' as it is usually performed at night. In this dance, male tambourine and bendir players group themselves in the centre of a circle formed by female dancers who dance round them.

During this festival, the women have the privilege of choosing a potential male partner. They take particular care of their appearance by dressing in their best finery and adorning themselves with exquisite local handcrafted silver jewellery. They also braid their hair. Special attention is paid to their facial tattoos, and decorative henna patterns are applied to their hands and feet. They use the henna patterns to identify the tribe they belong to and to ward off the 'evil eye' which is thought to bring bad luck.

For several days, the mountainside reverberates with the sounds of laughter, music, singing and hand clapping. At the closing of the Moussem, those lucky enough to have found a suitable partner are married by the Doul (notary). They then sing love songs and perform the Ahaidous, another popular dance from the region, this time originating from the Middle Atlas, in which men and women form a huge circle and beat out a rhythm by stamping their feet to the beat of the drums.

Although these dances of the Berbers which are performed in the valleys of the Atlas Mountains vary from tribe to tribe, there are many basic similarities. Many of the dances, such as the Ahaidous, for example, are reminiscent of those held at festivals in Crete and Greece. In most of these dances, dancers and musicians move round in circles or separate lines, drawing towards each other to dance face to face and shoulder to shoulder, then moving away. They continue to dance by repeating the sequence several times.

In a variant of the Ahaidous dance the participants perform in two long lines, with the women standing in front of the men clapping to the rhythm while dancing on the spot. During many of these dances the men will join the women in singing and chanting.

The Ahwas, a circle dance, begins with a solo artist singing the melody. There then follows a shout, a signal for the musicians to beat out the rhythm on their Bandirs which are large framed drums. The speed of the dance is determined by the male musicians who crouch inside a circle formed by the women. In turn, the women sing and clap their hands to the rhythm of the drums. As they move around in a circle, taking tiny, shuffling steps, they gently shimmy their shoulders from side to side. The dance reaches its climax as the musicians quicken the pace of the rhythm.

The Taskiouine is a virile and powerful dance of the warriors from the High Atlas, close to the Ouar Zazate.

Dressed in white tunics and with powder flasks on their shoulders, the warriors energetically beat out a pulsating rhythm with their feet, clap their hands and shake their shoulders simultaneously. The Tissant de Tatar or 'Dance of the Dagger', is performed south of Agadir by men and women dressed entirely in indigo blue who dance as though they were performing a rite.

The Taureg Nomads are the first Berber inhabitants of the Sahara Desert, originating from the southern area of Algeria in North Africa. These Muslim tribal people roam vast, harsh and inhospitable regions and are known as the 'People of the Veil' or 'Kel Tagilmus.' Although from age twenty-five onwards the men are veiled, the women remain unveiled. The veil, which is either black or a rich indigo blue, matches the robe they wear over white trousers, and is wrapped around their heads and faces so that only their eyes and the tips of their noses are exposed. This swathe of cloth, called a Tagilmus, is not worn for religious reasons but as protection from the harsh desert winds, sandstorms and exposure from the searing heat of the sun and extreme cold of the night.

Tuareg men are known for their bravery and skill as fighters, and for centuries wielded control over the hostile lands of the Sahara Desert. Their life is one of great hardship, as they act as herdsmen while roaming vast distances from the Ghadames in Libya, approximately 420 miles south of Tunis, and westwards through the Sahara to Tomouctou (Timbuktu). Their travelling lifestyle tends to isolate them from other Berber tribes.

These Berber people are also known as the 'blue people' because of an indigo blue dye which they use so frequently that it colours their skin. Over time, this dye impregnates the skin, and because they do not bathe regularly, the skin retains a permanent blue tinge, which the Tauregs consider beneficial.

Taureg women are much less restricted than women of

other tribes in Morocco. They enjoy a considerable amount of sexual freedom before marriage. Taureg women are described as being extremely lazy and are not expected to work. Much of their time is spent singing, dancing, doing needlework and composing poems relating to tribal life. Taureg women rarely marry beneath their status and are allowed to choose their own partners. A man marrying a woman of higher status improves his position within the society and if he marries out of his own tribe he is obliged to move over to that of his wife's.

Taureg women grease their hair and apply a great deal of make-up to their faces. Like women from other tribes, they wear henna on their fingers and toes. Taureg tribes have several social categories, ranging from the nobility to priests, slaves and serfs, who are ruled by a king. Ultimately, however, the hierarchy is based on a matriarchal system and the lineage is passed down in line through generations on the mother's side of the family.

The Guedra, a type of dance from the south of Morocco performed by the Tauregs, is a blessing dance. Rather than involving the exorcism of demons or spirits it is a purely joyful and spiritual experience, unlike other dances such as those of the Zar cult or the Hadraa. (The word 'Guedra' is also the name of a cooking pot covered with animal skins that has been converted into a drum that the Tauregs carry around with them.) The Guedra is an ancient ritual dance of pre-Islamic origin, which for a long time has been disliked by Islamic fundamentalists. Nevertheless, the dance has survived and is still performed today.

The Guedra begins with several men and women gathering in a circle around a woman dressed entirely in black who starts her performance in a kneeling position. Sometimes the dance is performed by an older woman of the tribe, with a younger woman moving rhythmically into a trance-like state induced by progressive drumming, hand clapping and chanting. The tempo of the claps and counter-claps, called 'rema' (claps to the beat), are performed to the constant rhythm of the drums. The chanting begins with continuous long chants, which escalate as the dance progresses. As the dance speeds up and reaches its climax, the singing changes to short, frenzied guttural screams. On occasion these dances have reportedly lasted up to three hours and more.

The original goal of the ancient dance was magical, intending to promote life and growth consisting of coitus movements such as the rolling and thrusting movements of the hips which were possibly for the purpose of sexual stimulation. As already discussed, centuries ago dance movements included the rotary movements of the hips and thrusting to and fro of the pelvis and abdominal activity and are evocative of the movements performed by dancers today. Erotic dances such as the belly dance are no longer pure peasant dances, as Curt Sachs surmises, 'If this path of seigniorial culture leads to the spectacular dance of the Oriental peoples, with the pure peasant dances we are already in the midst of the folk dance of the occident. For what survives today as the peculiar possession of the European 'folk' is for the most part merely the common property of that great peasant culture which since the high Stone Age has been held by all the planter peoples of Europe, Asia and Northern Africa.' (*World History of the Dance*, Curt Sachs, 1937.)

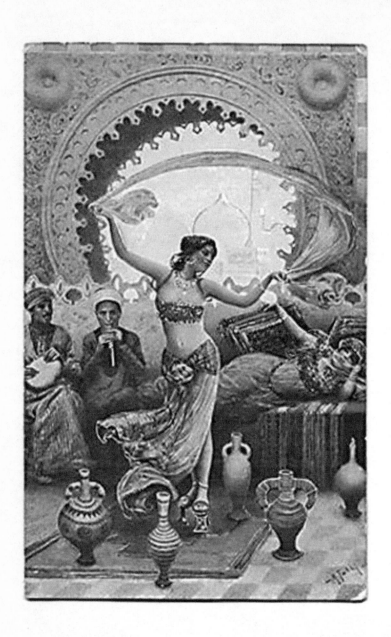

3

Music and Instruments of Ancient Times

As early belly dance styles would have been influenced by the type of instruments and music used in the Middle East throughout the pre-Christian era, this chapter will look at some of the earliest recorded means of music-making so that the reader gains a better understanding of the origins and development of belly dance. In this chapter we will therefore look to Ancient Egypt for a useful start point from which to understand the development of music throughout history, as evidence of instruments dating back to 3000 BCE and beyond is provided in the famous wall paintings of Egypt's many temples and tombs.

Music played an essential role in the life of the Ancient Egyptians, whatever the occasion. There was music on secular and religious processions, feast days, funerals and banquets, music for when they worked and played and music simply for pleasure. Music was regarded as a sacred art within the temples, where hymns were sung and dancers entertained in honour of their deities, accompanied by skilled musicians playing percussion and wind instruments.

During the time of the Old Kingdom (2686-2160 BCE), orchestras usually consisted of the oboe, shovel-shaped harp, end-blown flute and double clarinet. Vocal harmony, hand clapping, drums, clappers, rectangular tambourines and rattles provided the rhythm. One Old Kingdom relief from a tomb near Giza shows a basic ensemble of the time consisting of two harpists and two flautists, each with their own chironomist (*Complete Temples of Ancient Egypt*, Richard Wilkinson, 2000) who was a musician who used hand signals of unknown meaning, apparently to co-ordinate other musicians.

Most professional musicians were nubile young women, who were also employed as servants in the homes of the Egyptian nobility and the wealthy. In addition to their jobs as servants, they were frequently hired to entertain at banquets and other festivals (*Music and Musicians in Ancient Egypt*, Lise Manniche, 1991). Many formal banquets have been well documented on temple walls and monuments of the 18th Dynasty (1550-1295 BCE). The Opet Feast of Tutankamun is said to be one of the most impressive celebrations recorded by a king. It was immortalised on the walls of Luxor temple at the end of the 18th Dynasty and illustrates sacred and military performances, dancing and acrobatics. Guests attending a feast are depicted on the 18th Dynasty tomb of Nebamnun which is now in the British Museum (*Music and Musicians in Ancient Egypt*, Lise Manniche, 1991).

An elaborate representation of a banquet from the same tomb shows an ensemble of female musicians dressed in fine transparent clothing adorned with jewels and lotus blossoms. Sitting on their heads are cones of sweet, heady perfumed fat that would slowly melt and drip down their elegant coifed wigs as they entertained. Three of the musicians are standing together playing the oboe, lute and harp, while a second oboist sits with three others who are clapping their hands together to provide a rhythm as the dancers perform (*Music and Musicians of Ancient Egypt*, Lise Manniche, 1991).

Egyptians loved to drink large quantities of beer, known as 'hqt', and also wine at these lavish events and from the many tomb paintings depicting ancient 'party' scenes with guests being carried home in a drunken state it seems that becoming intoxicated was not necessarily considered shameful. They would also gorge themselves on a variety of game, meat, fruit, and sweet sticky cakes and sometimes indulged in a choice of no less than forty different types of bread. Whilst eating and drinking, they would be entertained by musicians playing harps, lutes and lyres, accompanying lithe young dancers whose movements varied from slow, sensuous movements to wild acrobatic stunts such as cartwheels, backbends and somersaults. In addition to the dancers and musicians, singers, acrobatic dwarfs and wrestlers were hired to provide further amusement.

In the wealthy homes of Ancient Egypt, while dinner was being prepared, guests would be warmly welcomed and entertained by singers and dancers, along with a group of musicians playing the lyre, tambourine, flute and an instrument classified as a guitar because of its flat back and curving sides (though it may not have much resembled the modern version). After the guests had eaten the entertainment would be resumed.

Around 2500 BCE, at Ur (now part of Iraq), the greatest city of Southern Chaldea, musicians were known to have been sacrificed and buried along with their instruments in royal tombs to accompany the dead to a life hereafter. Senmut, a most trusted servant of Hatshepsut and a great lover of music, had his minstrel buried with his harp not far from his own tomb. It must be said, however, that Egyptian tombs of the 1st Dynasty are believed to be the only ones with sacrificial burials (*Temples, Tombs and Hieroglyphs A Popular History of Ancient Egypt*, Barabara Mertz, 1990).

Unfortunately we can only guess the importance of the role of musicians and their instruments and wonder how they were played and sounded in magical and religious ceremonies and other festivities that were celebrated by Ancient Egyptians. There has been much speculation about whether or not the Egyptians developed musical notation, a system of symbols or figures. According to one expert, Hans Hickman, the chironomist could, by different hand positions, be dictating to the musicians which notes to play. The chironomist was usually a singer who presided over the group of musicians and singers and who made specific gestures towards the ensemble, possibly acting as a musical director, as illustrated on the tomb of Werirniptah, Saqqara (5th Dynasty), located in the British Museum (*Music and Musicians in Ancient Egypt*, Lise Manniche, 1991).

Dr. Lise Manniche, who is a Danish Egyptologist, makes an interesting comparison of Egyptian music with the classical music of Mauritania, which, although based on a complicated musical theory of modes, melodies and rhythm, is passed on from generation to generation orally. At the start of their performance, the musicians would have tuned into one of the modes of the melody the singer hummed to them. Thus the singer may perhaps have been likened to the chironomist. If the Egyptians had an oral tradition, rather than written notation, it is easy to see how such a tradition could easily be lost.

The oldest musical notation known had a scale of five tones and was constructed using a series of four of these scales. The notation was played on a twenty-two stringed harp, a commonplace instrument in Ancient Egypt and the later Mediterranean world. It is possible the Assyrians inherited this musical notation from the Babylonians (*Ancient Records of Egypt*, James Henry Breasted, 1906).

The earliest musical instrument used by ancient people recorded by Egyptian sources was the clapper, which evolved from a hunter's weapon - the 'throw stick' - similar in shape to a boomerang. It was an instrument from which the cymbals we use today most probably developed.

While lying in wait among the thickets of the tall papyrus reeds growing along the marshy banks of the River Nile in pursuit of water fowl, the hunters would strike their hunting sticks together to produce a sharp sound. This would startle their quarry and flush them out. The hunters would then hurl their sticks at the fowl as they took to the air in fright. Such hunting was a favourite leisure activity amongst the nobility in Egypt.

On occasion, these hunting sticks were transformed into percussion instruments, by being held in each hand and struck together to create a rhythmic sound. They were often played in an effort to help motivate the workers in the vineyards, as they picked and trod the grapes, and the farm labourers as they sowed and reaped the harvest. Workers would strike their sticks together as they followed each other in single file while taking long strides, in the hope that the magic striding dance would ensure a successful harvest (*World History of the Dance*, Curt Sachs, 1937).

Dancers depicted on the walls of tombs in 2000 BCE are seen to be playing clappers, as they performed in honour of Hathor the cow goddess. In the Middle Kingdom (2055-1650 BCE) clappers were either one-handed or two-handed and were struck against each other to create a rhythmic pattern. Usually they were made of wood or ivory and were approximately 10 to 15 inches (25 to 38 cm) in length. They were rounded on their outer side at one end. The insides were flat and the other ends were carved into the shape of a human hand, an animal, or the head of Hathor.

A pottery vessel made around 3500 BCE appears to illustrate clappers being played by female dancers at the Temple of Dendera (*El Amrah and Abydos*, D. Randall-Maciver & A. C. Mace, for the Egypt Exploration Fund 1902).

The cult rattle called the sistrum was a sacred magical percussion instrument used by the Ancient Egyptians. They used it in the ritual worship of gods and goddesses and it was shaken vigorously along with other noisy instruments. It was considered a great honour to hold a sistrum in the temples. (The goddess Hathor was often seen holding a sacred sistrum.) Its noisy rattling sound was used to chase away evil spirits who hated noise and it was known to be used by Bes, the ugly dwarf god, to soothe and protect women from harm during childbirth. In the tombs of Armana, from the New Kingdom (1550-1069 BCE), for example, there are wall paintings that depict gods like Bes and Tawaret, who are both connected with childbirth. During the 3rd Intermediate Period (1069-664 BCE) a number of magical figurines used to provide protection during childbirth and nourish the young typically show Bes, as a monkey, or a nude female sometimes holding a musical instrument or suckling (*Oxford History of Ancient Egypt*, Ian Shaw, 2000).

There were two types of sistrum. The older of the two was the Naos-shaped version, which appeared to resemble the shape of a miniature temple, and which dated back to the Old Kingdom (2686-2160 BCE). 'Naos' – which is an ancient Greek word referring to the innermost part of a temple, usually in the form of a rectangular box and often containing the divine image (*British Museum Dictionary of Ancient Egypt*, Ian Shaw and Paul Nicholson, 1995) – means 'house of the gods', that is, a Greek temple. These instruments were made from faience, a glazed composition made from powdered quartz coated with a vitreous paste. It was either blue or turquoise in colour, and when fired shone like polished glass. The Naos-shaped sistrum consisted of a handle shaped like a papyrus stem that supported a frame. Within this frame were two or three metal crossbars from which hung several small metal discs that produced a noisy, jingling, rattling sound when shaken.

The other type of sistrum was usually made of wood or metal and was adorned with either the carved cow's head of Hathor, who was said to favour the instrument, or with the figure of Bes, the dwarf god. Later, cats were added, during the period from around 650 to 27 BCE.

On the remains of a stone vase sculpted by Cretan artists, a procession of Cretan peasant farmers are shown carrying wooden pitchforks over their shoulders, accompanied by young people whose gender is not defined. Their mouths are wide open and they appear to be singing a harvest song, more than likely in honour of the earth mother in the belief that she would ensure the fertility of the land. A priest leads the group with his head shaven in the Egyptian fashion, carrying a sistrum in his upraised arm (*Ancient Records of Egypt*, James Henry Breasted, 1906).

The menat was a heavy beaded necklace consisting of several rows of beads made of faience, joined at the ends with a clasp, which was shaken by priestesses, queens and noble ladies when the sistrum was shaken. The menat-necklace was never described as a musical instrument, although it played an essential role in temple and funerary rituals. It was most often associated with the female temple personnel, as depicted in the relief from the temple of Sethos I at Abydos (*The Complete Temples of Ancient Egypt*, Richard H. Wilkinson, 2000). It was also linked to the concept of birth and rebirth. It is interesting to note that it can be seen worn around the neck of Hathor as she escorted Queen Nefertiti towards the throne of Osiris. Indeed, Hathor was regularly portrayed on the menat-counterpoise attached to necklaces worn by female dancers.

On a carving in the tomb of Ramose in Thebes (around 1350 BCE), started just as the young Amenhotep IV came to power, and discovered in 1860, women are shown with sistrums and menats. In a painting on the wall of Amenemhat at Thebes from around 1400 BCE and during the 18th Dynasty, three guests are shown shaking the menat-necklace during dances at a funery feast (*Music and Musicians of Ancient Egypt*, Lise Manniche, 1991).

Many instruments such as the lute, lyre, oboe and rectangular harp arrived in the New Kingdom (1550-1069 BCE) from Central Asia, along with skilled instrumentalists who had a profound influence on Ancient Egyptian people. Lutes had either a short or long neck though the latter was much preferred. These instruments were played together with boat-shaped harps and lyres, and may be seen on many Theban wall paintings of the 18th Dynasty. Only women played them.

Lutes are still used in Turkish and Arabic music. The short-necked oud or ud, the most widely available, is one of the most revered instruments in the Middle East and its players are highly regarded. In the 13th century (CE), the oud was adopted by Christians from Northern Spain from their Moorish Islamic neighbours, the Arab and Berber conquerors and occupants of Southern Spain. Throughout Europe, the use of the lute became widespread and the instrument was very popular in the later Middle Ages.

The izmar was, and still is, played exclusively by the young women of the Taureg tribes. It is an instrument usually played to accompany poets and singers at gatherings for those who are not yet betrothed. The instrument's body is made from half a dried pumpkin that has been hollowed out and covered with goatskin. The goatskin has two large holes in it and is attached to the shell of the pumpkin, either by small, sharp thorns or string. Its neck is made from a stick that is set at the upper end of the pumpkin.

The Kissar, a bowl-shaped member of the lyre family, was a stringed instrument made of tortoiseshell or wood known to exist in Ancient Egypt, Sudan and other areas of Western Africa before 200 BCE. The twelve string version dates back to 500 BCE and those with three or four strings date back as far as 900 BCE. This bowl-shaped lyre is believed to have existed in Ur and then to have spread to Assyria, Central Asia and Greece, where it was found illustrated on pottery vessels, its shape resembling that of a small harp. The bowl lyre was an accompaniment to poetry and ballads. More recently, it spread to the Sudan where it was called the El Tanbur (*The Sudanese Lyre or the Nubian Kissar*, Gwendolen Plumley, 1976). An early representation of the lyre is seen being played by a man of Semitic origin around 1900 BCE (*The History of Musical Instruments*, Curt Sachs, 1940).

Until around 2700 BCE, the lyre was unknown in Egypt but it played a very important role in ensembles during Sumerian ceremonies. It was not until several centuries later that a painter (name unknown) depicted the lyre in the Nile Valley, illustrating a lyricist and his fellow travellers on their way to Egypt. The Middle Kingdom (2055-1650 BCE) saw further importation of both lyre and lute. That the lyre first appears in tomb paintings in the hands of foreigners or Boudins, rather than in the hands of Egyptians, is well illustrated, according to the contemporary historian Douglas Irvine (*Ancient Egypt Magazine*, 2001), by the famous painting of the lyre player from Beni Hassan, dated around 1850 BCE. Lyres are still widely used today in Africa, Ethiopia, Etrea and the Sudan, where they are known as tamburas. Sumerian and Mesopotamian lyres have either long or short necks and are shown alongside the souffra or alamiya, an end-blown flute, also used in the cult of the Zar for a trance dance performed by women to exorcise evil spirits.

Lyres were first depicted on Sumerian art works of about 3000 BCE and were asymmetrical. They rested vertically on the ground and stood higher than someone seated. The shorter arm of the yoke was held close and the longer arm away from the player. These lyres consisted of eight to eleven strings that were plucked in a way similar to that of the harp, with both hands and without the use of a plectrum. Syrian lyres were smaller and lighter, and these were plucked with a plectrum. (*History of Musical Instruments*, Curt Sachs, 1940).

According to Curt Sachs, flutes, like bone scrapers (notched instruments that the player scrapes with a rigid object to create a sound), are phallic. Our ancestors could not overlook the resemblance of this instrument to the penis. Sachs states that even in modern occidental slang, the penis is designated by flute names. Early civilisations connected flute playing with phallic ceremonies, fertility and rebirth rites.

The oblique, an end-blown flute, is made from a piece of bamboo, like a tube, that has about three or four finger holes. The instrument has no mouthpiece but is played by blowing across its upper edge. This particular type of flute has been found in many regions of the world, which suggests its invention may not have originated from one particular source. The oblique has changed very little since it was played in orchestras of the Old Kingdom (2686-2160 BCE), where it appears to have been played exclusively by men.

Lise Manniche (*Music and Musicians of Ancient Egypt*, 1991) lists its appearance in tomb chapels of the Middle Kingdom (2055-1650 BCE) at Meir, one of which shows the first representation of a woman playing this instrument. It is interesting to note that the two flautists shown on a tomb at Giza are playing different types of flute. While one flute is being held obliquely, the other is held horizontally, which may suggest that the horizontal flute is of the uffatah type, being shorter and having a wider bore than that of the nay. Or that it is in fact a double clarinet that is shown in profile. Antefoker's tomb at Thebes 1950 BCE depicts a female flautist accompanied by a woman who appears to be a chironomist.

Egyptian flutes cut from cane were smaller than many primitive ceremonial flutes. They were about a yard (one metre) long and half an inch (1.3 cm) wide, and had between two and six finger holes near the lower end. An excavated flute shows a thumbhole in the back. In the latter part of the

7th century (CE), when the Arabs had conquered Morocco, the size of the lute was reduced and replaced by a heavy oblong body with a smaller pear-shaped or hemispherical body (half round), with strings attached to lateral pegs.

In 1999, David Derbyshire reported in the UK newspaper the *Daily Mail* on a major scientific discovery of a perfectly preserved neolithic flute that had been buried since 7000 BCE in Jiahu, a province of China. This flute, the oldest working instrument ever to have been found, is about one foot (30.5 cm) long and was made from the bone of a bird. It has seven main holes, plus two smaller holes towards the end of the bone, and through tonal analysis of the flute it seems the tones and scales are remarkably similar to those of the western eight-note scale (*EurekeAlert! Magazine*,1999). Vertical flutes were first recorded in the 4th millennium BCE on a prehistoric slate that shows a hunter playing a flute to lure game.

In many instances flutes have been found next to human remains during the excavation of ancient tombs (*History of Musical Instruments*, Curt Sachs, 1940). These did not necessarily belong to musicians, as flutes were probably placed in tombs as life charms. Young boys played the flute as they climbed the steps to the top of pyramids, where priests would cut out their hearts and offer them to the sun. There is also evidence, such as the painting from the tomb of Kahif, the tomb-owner at Giza, that during the Middle Kingdom (2055-1650 BCE) flautists would often play their instruments in the fields under the shade of olive trees during leisure breaks when harvesting (*Music and Musicians of Ancient Egypt*, Lise Manniche, 1991).

At the end of the Middle Kingdom, flutes disappeared from banquet ensembles as did the shovel-shaped harps, but re-emerged in ritual music. Although the flute ceased to be represented in banquet ensembles after the Middle Kingdom, it retained its popularity and is still used today in North Africa as well as in other regions of the world.

The nay, the name of which came from Persia, is a reed instrument that is very similar to the end blown flute. Just under three feet (one metre) long and with a diameter of between half to seven-tenths of an inch (1.5 to 1.8 cm), it has six finger holes, and underneath, half way down its length, there is a thumbhole. The shorter, fatter version is just under 16 inches (40 cm), and about three-quarters of an inch (2 cm) in diameter. It has between four and eight holes and is closer in style to the modern uffatah (a shorter version of the flute with wider bores) whereas the modern version of the nay has only six holes. A tomb chapel of the Middle Kingdom (2055-1650 BCE) at Meir shows a woman playing the nay in the tomb of Amenemhat I's vizier, Antefoker, at Thebes 12th Dynasty (1950 BCE).

The material used for these instruments varies. Three flutes, which can be seen in a collection at the British Museum, are made of reed wood and bronze. The wooden flute has a bronze terminal fitting and the bronze flutes are inscribed with a demotic inscription dating to the Ptolemaic Period (approximately 332 BCE to 30 BCE).

In the Maghreb, which is the name given to the North African states of Morocco, Algeria, Tunisia, Mauritania and Libya (meaning 'sunset' in Arabic), the 'nay' is used as a solo instrument in the ritual dance of the whirling dervishes. The origins of the dervishes can be traced to the 13th century Ottoman Empire, and they are infamous for the whirling dance they perform to induce a state of divine ecstasy. It is a popular instrument in ensembles and is used in classical music throughout the Islamic world.

Another popular reed instrument in ancient times was the double clarinet that was played exclusively by men in the Old Kingdom (2686-2160 BCE). It consisted of two parallel pipes of equal lengths, tied together with strips of cloth secured with resin. Musicians depicted on reliefs are shown holding the instrument in a horizontal position and covering the same holes on both pipes while playing. It is thought that as the two pipes were never exactly alike in pitch, the sound would not have been in unison but slightly out of tune. When played, according to pictorial depictions, the entire mouthpiece of the double reed clarinet was held in the mouth of the player. Since no mouthpieces have survived, however, we can only surmise the type of reed used. The double reed clarinet has been assumed to be similar to the zumar of today. This has a mouthpiece consisting of a tube of narrow reed, flattened at the top with a tongue cut into it that forms the vibrating reed. A tomb chapel of the Middle Kingdom (2055-1650 BCE) at Meir shows a woman playing the nay in the tomb of Amenemhat I's vizier, Antefoker, at Thebes (1950 BCE, 12th Dynasty).

Wind instruments of Middle Eastern origin are still played throughout the whole of the Islamic world. Double clarinets have existed for around 5000 years and many are of the same design as those excavated from Egyptian tombs of the 1st century BCE. These single-reed instruments are always found in pairs and are made of cane. Three slits are cut into the upper end of the cane that is held in the mouth and blown to present a musical note.

Oboes arrived in the New Kingdom (1550-1069 BCE) from Central Asia, along with lutes and lyres. These instruments were also used by priests during ritual ceremonies, including burials. Double oboes were recorded as of 2800 BCE. They had two pipes of unequal length so that the longer pipe was used to play notes that the shorter pipe couldn't hit. Double oboes were made up of two pieces of thin reed or cane about two feet long and bound together at either end with thread or string. It had a mouthpiece of two rushes which were inserted into the upper end of each tube.

Finger holes were at the front of the instrument and some double oboes also had thumb holes. When played they were either held almost parallel or at an angle. The sound was described as penetrating and rather shrill (*History of Musical Instruments*, Curt Sachs, 1940).

The mizmar was a wind instrument of the Ancient Egyptians. Originally made of metal with a cylindrical funnel, it was splayed bell-like at one end and cup-shaped at the mouthpiece. Two such instruments, both bell-shaped, were found in Tutankhamen's tomb that differ slightly in shape, from the more slender that gradually splays out, to something shorter and wider.

The more slender of the two was made from beaten silver with a gold mouthpiece, with its bell decorated with a golden band. The shorter was made from bronze or copper and had a silver mouthpiece. Its lower and upper ends were overlaid with gold, while the middle section was of black ebony. Skilled metal workers from Mosul in Iraq, a city built on the banks of the River Tigris, were masters at inlaying silver on bronze and brass, and were renowned for their precision and skills in such techniques. Mizmars have a powerful tone, which sounds very similar to our modern trumpets. Plutarch, a Greek historian, likened the blare of the instrument to an ass's bray but I am not sure that trumpet enthusiasts would entirely agree with his statement! Mizmars were used in sacred and secular ceremonies and were represented on reliefs of the temple of Queen Hatshepsut at Deir el Bahari. No mizmars are believed to have survived before the New Kingdom (1550-1069 BCE), except for the two mentioned above that were discovered in Tutankhamen's tomb. However, instruments similar to the nafir, a Moroccan trumpet, have been found. They produced a single note when blown, usually during wedding processions.

A damaged relief of a boating scene from the Old Kingdom

(2686-2160 BCE) shows a young boy holding two decoy birds and blowing into a tube (*Music and Musicians in Ancient Egypt*, Lise Manniche 1991). This object has been tentatively described by historians as a trumpet and is believed to be one of the earliest examples of a trumpet discovered.

In 1415 BCE trumpets were first pictured being played by soldiers. Standard bearers and trumpeters of Mustansir, a caliph of the Abbasid dynasty, administered from Baghdad (749–1258 CE) were depicted playing trumpets in a miniature painting of 1237 CE heralding the end of Ramadan and the start of a feast celebrated at the end of the Islamic holy week. (*Music and Musical Instruments in the World of Islam*, Jean Jenkins and Poul Rovsing Olsen 1976; *The Last Two Million Years*, Readers Digest Association 1973.)

Apart from its military purpose, the trumpet was a sacred instrument played to honour Osiris, King of the Dead and Lord of Resurrection, who loved to dance and enjoy the sound of music. The military function, apart from warfare, was to entertain during processions worshipping the gods, in the streets of the towns and cities and sometimes within the palace walls. The drums were played by the Nubians, who were usually accompanied by women shaking the sistrum, playing the clappers or blowing trumpets.

Although most of the percussionists of Ancient Egypt we have information about were women (*When the Drummers Were Women*, Layne Redmond, 1997) male percussionists appear as military drummers. The type of drum that was used by the military had a barrel-shaped body with a membrane laced into position at either end of the barrel by leather thongs. When played, the drum was suspended from around the neck by a cord and was held either in a horizontal position or at an angle whilst being beaten by both hands to create a rhythm.

A well-preserved example of this type of drum was found

in a Middle Kingdom tomb at Beni Hassan, now in the Cairo Museum. A relief on mortuary walls of the Temple of Ramesses III from the New Kingdom (1550-1069 BCE), also shows drums and trumpets being played by the military, who were providing music for a feast in honour of the fertility god Min at Thebes. On a relief at Luxor temple, a drummer is drumming the beat to encourage those pulling a boat to synchronise their movements.

Drums in the Middle East today are varied and made from either wood or clay. A vase-shaped hand drum called the darabuka or tabla has one skin, and is held under the arm or suspended from a cord that rests over the shoulder of the musician. When played, the drum is beaten with both hands. The sounds differ according to how and where the drum is struck by the hands, whether in the middle or towards the edge. The darabuka seems to have originally entered Egypt during the invasion of a Western Asiatic people known as the Hyksos.

Excavations at Avaris in the Nile Delta have uncovered a set of three drums in the form of clay vases which would have had a membrane stretched over the drum at one end with the lower end left open. But this type of drum was rarely depicted, even in the New Kingdom (1550-1069 BCE). In Turkey such a 'goblet' drum is known as the dumbeleck and is played both in folk and classical music. In Iran this type of goblet drum called the 'dombak'. (The word 'dombalak' is a Pahlavian word from the Middle Persian language of the Sasanid Period.)

In the early kingdoms around the Great Lakes of Africa, an area known now as Central Uganda which was inhabited by a tribe known as Buchwezi, drums were used for accompanying dancers in ritual cults. Royal drums symbolised the supremacy of the king, and the larger the drum he possessed the more magical power he believed it gave him when communicating with his ancestors. These instruments were always kept in shrines and protected by especially chosen people, which may be the reason that some have survived today.

Women of the Taureg tribes hit drums to accompany the men when stick dancing and to find women beating huge drums in North African countries is not uncommon. For these women, the drum, which has a low, resonated sound, is a symbol of their femininity, motherhood and the earth mother.

Frame drums come in various sizes and are either round or rectangular. They consist of a frame in which miniature cymbals are inserted. Over the frame a single skin is stretched, which is beaten by hand to create a rhythm. The most well known drums are the duf, sometimes used today in Sufi or Dervish music, and the tambourine that is also known as the tar or bendir, which is an Arab term, is still played in some parts of the Middle East.

Rectangular tambourines were used at about the same time as boat-shaped harps, and such instruments can be seen on a relief from a building of Akhenaten in the New Kingdom around 1365 BCE. This shows women beating rectangular tambourines as they trekked through the woods, possibly to scare away birds and animals, or to ferret them out and drive them towards hunters hiding in the undergrowth. A unique specimen of a rectangular tambourine was found at Thebes in the burial ground of Senmut's mother. (Senmut was the favourite of Hatshepsut and the architect of Deir el Bahari.) In the New Kingdom (1550-1069 BCE) women often used these instruments in ceremonial and religious ceremonies, though it was not unknown for priests to play them on some occasions – especially as the round tambourine increased in popularity towards the end of the New Kingdom as shown by many scenes depicted on temples of the time.

Bes, the dwarf god, was often portrayed as a musician. On many reliefs he can be seen dancing and playing various instruments, including the tambourine and drum, in secular rituals. Bes is also depicted on furniture that was found in the Tomb of Queen Tiy's parents, Yuya and Tuyu, in the 18th Dynasty. Queen Tiy was one of Amenhotep III's (1390–1352 BCE) many wives, who, along with her daughter Satamun, bore the title of 'Great Royal Wife' during the 18th Dynasty (*Oxford History of Ancient Egypt*, Ian Shaw, 2000). Here, Bes is depicted striking a frame drum, and in scenes on other temple walls is playing the same instrument in honour of his mistress Hathor some 1,000 years later.

Crotals were a type of miniature bell, possibly the oldest recorded, consisting of a small perforated sphere, usually metal, inside of which were loose jangling pellets (*Michigan State University*, 2003). Miniature cymbals attached to a pair of handles, were used during rituals in the Middle Kingdom (2055–1650 BCE) and cymbals from pharaonic civilisations have been found in various sizes. It was thought they were played by the goddess Isis and her sister Nephthys. In the Middle Kingdom, they may have travelled from Western Asia to Greece along with the orgiastic cult of Cybele, the Phrygian goddess of nature and Dionysus, the god of fertility, ecstasy and wine. Cymbals were considered to reflect unconstrained debauchery and effeminate life according to writers of the 3rd century BCE, such as Athenaeus (*Music and Musicians of Ancient Egypt*, Lise Manniche, 1991). A pair of such cymbals found in the temple of Amon around the 1st century BCE is now held in the British Museum.

Small finger cymbals known as zills (in Turkey) or zagats (across the Arab world) are widely played during Turkish and Egyptian celebrations by belly dancers when entertaining in night clubs, restaurants or at other functions such as weddings. These are metal discs with a wide, flat brim and a concave centre that resonates when struck together. They come in sets of four and are worn on the middle finger and thumb of each hand, around the base of the nail, secured by an elastic strap.

They are usually played by a musician or a dancer to provide musical accompaniment that is created by striking them together to produce a bell-like ring.

In Turkey, finger snapping involving the use of both hands is sometimes used as a rhythmic accompaniment for belly dancers rather than cymbals.

The oldest and most coveted instrument of the Ancient Egyptians was the harp. The arched harp was closely related to the Sumerian harp and although it has not yet been established whether it was brought from Sumer to Egypt or vice-versa, musicologists think that it probably came from Sumer (*History of Musical Instruments*, Curt Sachs, 1940). Sumer, now Southern Iraq, emerged around 3500 BCE. and had developed large cities by the 4th millennium, whereas Egyptians of the same period were living in much smaller communities or villages (*Ancient Egypt*, Paul Johnson 1978).

In the Pharaonic Period, the harp's shallow sound box resembled the shape of a shovel. Egyptian harps were vertical and stood at a height of seven feet. (2.13 metres) They were placed on the ground and played by harpists in a sitting or kneeling position. Painting of harps have been found on numerous reliefs over a period of 3,000 years, including on the tomb of Ramesses III of the 20th Dynasty who reigned from 1184-1153 BCE which depicts a harp standing at a vertical height of seven feet (*British Museum Dictionary of Archaeology*, Ian Shaw and Paul Nicholson, 1995).

Arched harps have only been discovered in Sumer; none have been found in Mesopotamia after the Sumerian epoch. Around 2000 BCE in Egypt they were gradually replaced by angular harps that came from Asia. These had many more strings and were taller and heavier, which enabled the harpist to stand erect when playing. Although the sizes of harps varied greatly, the basic design remained much the same as the original version, consisting of a gently curved neck leading to a shallow sound box which was covered by a skin. This type of harp had between six and twelve strings that were fastened to small pegs at the neck on each end of the instrument, and a suspension rod, which was fixed into the sound box shoulder.

In secular musical performances, portable harps were mostly used by male blind harpists who sang songs of love, life and death and accompanied dancers when entertaining. Many male harpists wore blindfolds, but whether harpists were generally blind is debatable. At Tell el Amarna in the tombs of officials, male palace musicians are depicted wearing blindfolds while performing. It is not certain what this signified (*Music and Musicians in Ancient Egypt*, Lise Manniche, 1991).

In the Middle Kingdom (2055-1650 BCE) the ladle-shaped harp was well represented on tombs at Thebes, a religious centre for over 1,000 years. This harp varied in design, had between seven and eleven strings and became an instrument used by solo artists. The earliest reliable representation of the ladle harp is illustrated on two wall paintings in the New Kingdom tomb of Inene, early 18th Dynasty. The portable-shaped harp was popular with both sexes and was used on secular occasions. It is illustrated being played by a woman on a tomb in Thebes of Nebamun in the 18th Dynasty.

A harp known as the boat-shaped harp of the Middle Kingdom era was discovered in a tomb at Beni Hasan and has been preserved in a Liverpool museum. It became very popular in ensembles and was played by both men and women.

Male and female harpists are frequently shown playing together in the company of singers or chironomists. One 12th Dynasty painting from the tomb of Anefoker, 1950 BCE, shows a male and female harpist performing together on very similar instruments. On another scene from the same tomb, two shovel-shaped harps are shown that vary in size and are being played by a man and a woman. The woman plays the smaller of the harps, as it rests on her knee rather than on the ground. Both harps are skilfully decorated around their necks; the woman's harp with a female head and that of the male with the head of a falcon. At the time of the Old Kingdom, the harp was mostly played by men; however, depictions on the tomb of Mereruka in Saqqara do show women playing harps (*Music and Musicians in Ancient Egypt*, Lise Manniche, 1991).

Another instrument that originated in the Middle East was the dulcimer, also known as the santir, which is derived from the Greek word 'psalterion'. This instrument is known to have existed in Persia and Central Asia, and is believed to have been brought to North Africa and Spain by Arabs. It is still used today in Turkish classical music. It consists of a wooden frame with a number of strings stretched over it. The strings are struck by hand-held hammers to create a musical sound.

Similar instruments known as zithers or qanoons were originally instruments of the Phoenicians and are known to have existed in Palestine, Syria and Persia (but not in either Egypt or Assyria). Zithers are mentioned in one of the older stories of the 'Arabian Nights', the famous volume of Arabian tales which were translated by Sir Richard Burton in 1850 and first appeared in Arabic in written form around 850 BCE (though the origins of these tales owe much to the storytelling cultures of India and Persia as well as the Arab world).

Two examples of zithers from the South East Palace at Nimrod in Assyria are carved on an exquisite ivory pyxis (little boxes or caskets) of the 8th century BCE. They were at first believed to be Assyrian instruments until definitely established as Phoenician. The forty strings of each zither are stretched across a flat, trapezoid-shaped box (a flattened down rectangular shape). Music is then produced by plucking the strings with a plectrum and, depending on the size, the instrument is played either on the knee of the musician or on a flat surface.

From evidence of musical scenes depicted on many representations discovered over the centuries on temple walls and on the tombs of the pharaohs, kings and queens of Ancient Egypt, it is apparent that from the Middle Kingdom (2055-1650 BCE) onwards Egyptian musicians used instruments that were fairly similar to those of our own. As opposed to the simple bells and ivory clappers depicted on pre-dynastic pottery vessels of the mid-4th millennium BCE during the New Kingdom the depiction of musical activities seems to have gained a new lease of life. In paintings of musical ensembles, new instruments joined the harp; double oboes, lutes, lyres, and trumpets appear also (*British Museum Dictionary of Ancient Music*, Ian Shaw and Paul Nicholson, 1995).

The Ancient Egyptian instruments were divided into four basic types:

Idiophones:	clappers, sistra, cymbals, bells (associated primarily with religious worship)
Membranophones:	tambourines (used by dancing girls at banquets), drums (for military purposes)
Aerophones:	flute, double clarinet and oboe, trumpet
Condophones:	harp, lute and lyre

Egyptians also had an instrument that resembled the guitar and consisted of two parts, a handle that was nearly three times the length of the body or a long flat neck, and an oval shaped hollow body. The instrument was made entirely of wood or covered with parchment. The upper surface was perforated with holes which allowed the sounds to escape. Three strings of catgut were stretched over the whole length of the body of the instrument, secured at the upper end by pegs, or passed through openings in the handle and then bound and secured by knotting. At the lower end of the instrument the strings were fastened to a triangular piece of wood or ivory. It was struck by a plectrum that was attached by a cord to the neck. It was played equally by men or women who usually stood as they played it. Women also danced whilst playing. (*The Ancient Egyptians: Their Life and Customs*, J. Gardiner Wilkinson, 1853.)

Throughout the bible there are multiple references to music being played at celebrations to liven up events and encourage merry-making. The Hebrew word for feast, 'Hay', also means dance and God himself is recorded in the Bible as giving specific commands to the Israelites regarding how to celebrate, advising that they choose an unblemished lamb to sacrifice and blow the trumpet (or shofar). The Jewish prophet Isaiah, who lived between 740-650 BCE, described such events as follows: 'They have harps and lyres at their banquets, tambourines, flutes and wine.' (*The Living Past*, Ivar Lissner, 1957.)

After the Israelites had crossed the Red Sea, having made their escape from Egypt after many long years of slavery, Miriam, the prophet and sister of Moses and Aaron, led them in celebration. She took the timbrel, an oriental tambourine or tabor, in her hand and danced, which soon encouraged other women to participate and follow her.

Even when saying farewell, music was a cause for celebration. When, for example, Jacob left without saying a word to his father-in-law Laban, the elder caught up with him and said, 'Why did you flee secretly and trick me and did not tell me, so that I might have sent you away with mirth and songs, with tambourine and lyre?' (Exodus 15:201 Genesis 31:27).

Music that came from Persia and Byzantium to Arabia persisted for many centuries, reaching its peak during the 8th and 9th centuries (CE), particularly in the Islamic towns of Medina and Mecca, two famous Islamic religious centres. The music was very much patronised by the Arabs. Those who were wealthy made a business of buying male and female slaves whom they educated to sing and play musical instruments to a high standard. They would then re-sell and export them as entertainers.

Over the last 3000 years, despite numerous invasions and the threat from Christianity, Middle Eastern and North African music and instruments have survived and are now enjoying a revival in the West. We know that from before the Pharaonic Period up to the present, many musical instruments have changed little in sound or from their original appearance. In some instances they have even retained their original names.

Thanks to painstaking research carried out by Egyptologists, archaeologists, historians and musicologists, we have been given invaluable insights into the musical past and skills of ancient civilisations. This has helped us to understand the importance of the role music played throughout the lives of these ancient civilisations, and its ever-enriching influence on more modern times.

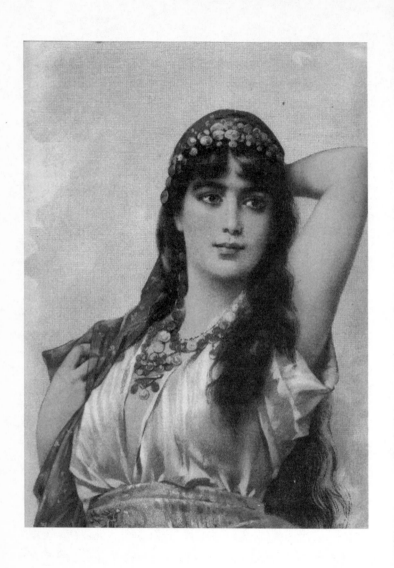

4

Gypsy Dances and Belly Dance

The belly dance, which has survived for thousands of years and is believed to be the oldest form of dance, evolved from the worship of the great mother goddess and is associated with child birth rituals. Belly dance grew out of a combination of fertility cults, religious rituals, magic and secular dances in ancient civilisations inextricably linked to the mother goddess cult. In the early 1920s, Armen Ohanian, an Armenian dancer from the Caucasus, described the belly dance as a birth ritual, stating that it is a 'dance of mystery and pain of motherhood'.

Over the centuries, music and dance have evolved in various forms, beginning with folk dances and the dances of migrating gypsies, who are believed to have travelled from the northern regions of India to the rest of the world. There is little doubt that these gypsies were largely responsible for the spread of oriental influences in dance and music that survived over the centuries through the intermix of complex Asian rhythms with dance styles of other countries.

There is much debate about when and why these people left their homeland and concerning which routes they followed on their travels. Although their lives are shrouded in mystery, as very little of their history or achievements were recorded, some progress in tracing their history has been made during the last two centuries in spite of the lack of documentary evidence available.

It has been claimed that the first migration of gypsies was around the early 13th century, during the period of the great warrior Genghis Khan, who established a Mongol empire that stretched from the Pacific to the Black Sea. This first migration was followed by a second in the 14th century, when the gypsies were persecuted and banished from India by Tamerlane (Timur-Lane) a tough Mongolian warrior who led his troops into Persia, Asia Minor and Syria, which he brutally ravaged between the years 1395 to 1400 CE.

This claim is disputed, however, as others believe that the gypsies migrated to Spain long before the 9th century, infiltrating the country as camp followers of the invading Muslim forces. Another theory is that a mass exodus of gypsies from Northern India to the Middle East began in the 10th century, where they settled and traded as metal workers, tradesmen and mercenaries, and also earned a living as minstrels, dancers, singers and fortune tellers.

Wherever gypsies settled they were, and still are, known by different names. Those settling in Russia are known as the Zignani and in Persia and Turkey as the Zingarri. Spanish gypsies are still known today as Gitanos and those from Northern Spain as Hungaros. In Germany they are called Zigeuner, in Hungary, Czigany and in France, Bohemians (*The Zincali: An Account of The Gypsies of Spain*, George Borro, 1996). The name for gypsies from the Netherlands is Gyptenaers, from Greece, Yifti and from Albania, Evgit. However, it is supposed that all these names derived from the term 'Zincali', meaning 'black men of the Zend'.

Eastern Influences on Spanish Dance

The Iberian Peninsula, that is, Spain and Portugal, was occupied in parts by settlers, believed to be travellers from

Africa, who integrated with Celtic tribes from the North.

Between 1100 and 509 BCE, the peninsular was invaded by the Phoenicians, Greeks, Carthaginians and Romans. Then, around the year 202 BCE, war broke out between the Romans and the Carthaginians and the latter were driven from the peninsular. The Romans then had the difficult task of pacifying the volatile Iberian tribes before they succeeded in making the area a single political state, which encompassed an area of thousands of miles from Cadiz to the Pyrenees

The Peninsula then became known as Hispania and its people the Hispano-Romans, adopted the cultural heritage of Rome, making Latin their common language, from which the Spanish language later evolved.

In approximately 712 CE the entire peninsula (apart from the mountainous northern regions, where the inhabitants managed to maintain their Christian identity) was invaded by Muslim armies, who reached the peninsular by crossing the Straits of Gibraltar from Africa. A new province was created called Anduylas or Al-Andalus (Andalucia), whose original name was said to have come from the Vandals, one of the peoples who inhabited the area, as 'Vandalus' means 'Lane of the Vandals.'

For several centuries, Spain was divided between the Moors, a blanket term describing Muslim conquerors and rulers in Andalucia between 711 and 1492 CE and the Christians.

The Moors, Berbers (the indigenous peoples of North Africa) and Arabs were hated and persecuted like the gypsies by the Spanish Christians. They were strictly forbidden to speak in Arabic or practice the rites of Islam. In 1492 the Moors were defeated by the Spanish and, along with the Jews, were banished from Spain. After seven centuries of Muslim presence, Spain emerged as the most powerful country in Europe, gaining control of the Americas following Columbus' discovery of the continent in 1492 and creating a vast empire. The first global age for the Spanish Empire lasted from around 1400–1600 CE. Spain's powerful rule in the US lasted little more than a century, however. The riches gained from Spanish America were recklessly squandered and the country rapidly declined.

Upheaval followed as Spain's rulers retreated into strict religious Roman Catholic orthodoxy and reactionary politics. Any opposition to the harsh regime or challenge by those who saw the ideals of liberalism as the only hope for Spain's recovery was ruthlessly opposed. In the 19th century, Spain began to emerge from the conflicts between Catholic conservatism and liberalism, which culminated in the civil war of 1936–9.

Around 1447, a great number of gypsies reached the Anatolian Plateau at the foot of the Pontic Mountains in Tukey, and Andulasia in Spain, an area that has been renowned for possessing a lively and colourful variety of music and folk songs. Whether the migrants travelled from the North to the Iberian Peninsula or came from the South over the Straits of Gibraltar to reach Spain is still very unclear.

Wherever the gypsies settled they were classed as outsiders, and hostility and prejudice towards them prevailed. Nowhere were they despised more than in Spain. Both the Spanish and the Moors looked upon the gypsies as the dregs of society. They were described as filthy, useless, godless and evil. The unwelcome gypsy migrants colonised Spanish towns and villages, creating gypsy quarters called 'Gitaneria', and plied their trades as horse dealers, blacksmiths, metal workers, knife sharpeners, peddlers, fortune tellers and minstrels. Among them were thieves, fraudsters and notorious robbers who viciously attacked and sometimes murdered defenceless travellers for their valuables. The female gypsies outside of their own society were regarded as loose women who, as a means of making a living, combined prostitution and dance, and sang filthy songs that violated all boundaries of common decency.

In 1499, laws were issued in Spain against the gypsies in a vain attempt to control their daily lives and criminal activities by preventing them from leaving their towns and villages. Not only were they ordered to find a taskmaster to serve but they had to convert to Christianity. If they failed to abide by these laws, they were severely punished or ordered to leave Spain. It was not only the gypsies who were forced to convert to Christianity; the same laws applied to Jews and Muslims who also faced exile from Spain if they failed to convert.

Although Jews and Muslims expressed a mutual dislike for the gypsies, when they, too, were expelled from Spain, all parties reluctantly coexisted and eventually united against their common enemy in a bid to survive in the dry, rough mountainous terrain to which they had been banished.

Until the late 1700s, numerous laws and royal edicts in Spain continued to be enforced in a bid to suppress and persecute the gypsies. They were forbidden to dress in the costumes of their choice or speak their own Romany language, visit trade fairs, or seek employment apart from farm labouring. They were also prohibited from owning livestock and even horses though they were allowed to keep mules. Penalties for breaking these laws constituted anything from two months to six years imprisonment, or permanent banishment from Spain. In spite of centuries of chastisement and terrible persecution, however, gypsies have managed to survive and continue to live successfully in many areas of Spain. They have also preserved their traditional dances, music and songs that have become part of the tapestry of Spain.

The Fandango goes back to before the 17th century and is said to have been primarily of Moorish influence, although there is little evidence to support this theory. It became established as an Andulasian folk dance that spread across from the South to many regions of Spain. As a result many regional variations were adopted, particularly in the provinces of Helva in the West and in Granada.

As the Spanish Fandango seen in the Basque provinces was so similar to that of the dancing style of the Ghawazee, this suggests the dance was introduced into Spain by the Arabs.

The Gaditans, the legendary female dancers from Gades, a province of Spain now known as Cadiz in Baetica, were very famous for their performances. The Roman poet and writer of epigrams, Marcus Valerius Martial (43-104 CE) wrote of them:

'Tireless the lustful move
In gentle tremor eager limbs.'
(*World History of the Dance*, Curt Sachs, 1937.)

In Cadiz the dance progressed and developed into a fine art form that became respected and acceptable entertainment. The Fandango greatly impressed the Romans, who invaded and took over Cadiz.

A tale about the Fandango, supposedly written in the 17th century, tells of the pope who heard that the dance was outrageous and recommended that it be immediately banned and that those who continued to dance it should be excommunicated. A cardinal, however, thought the offenders ought to have a chance to defend themselves. He interceded on behalf of the dancers who were given the chance to defend themselves by performing the Fandango for the clergy. One witness of the occasion reported:

'Their grace and vitality soon drove the frowns from the rows of the fathers whose souls were stirred by the lively emotion and strange pleasure. One by one their Eminencies began to beat time with their hands and feet, then suddenly the hall became a ballroom; as they sprang up, dancing the steps, and imitating the gestures of the dancers.' (Saint Basil Bishop of Caesarea.)

Following this exhibition, the Fandango was fully pardoned and restored to its former honour.

There is much dispute about the origins of the Flamenco, which remain mysterious. One theory is that the dance evolved from ancient sacred Hindu dances; another that it was introduced directly or indirectly by the gypsies who migrated from North Africa and India about the year 1400 CE. Another theory put forward is that it was brought to Andulasia in Spain by Iberians and Jews around the 8th century, who incorporated their complex Indian rhythms with Arabic melodies and combined their style of traditional dances with Spanish dancing. Juvenal, a Roman poet, referred to the Cadiz girls of Rome as 'Puellae Gaditanae', which means 'Dancing Girls from Gadir' who performed dances with bronze castanets during Emperor Trajan's reign. Domingo Manfredi, a Flamencologist and poet of the 1960s, claims that this was evidence enough to date the Flamenco back to classical times.

Others, however, have made the point that if the dance had come solely from the gypsies, then why did it not develop in all the other regions of the world in which gypsies settled? According to Cabaccero Bonaco in his book on Andulasian Dance, Flamenco is originally Andulasian and became influenced by Asiatic and Arab dances that eventually merged with gypsy dances that had been handed down from generation to generation.

Some theorists argue that Flamenco developed solely from Andulasia and was totally unaffected by outside influences. However, this idea has been strongly opposed by others who maintain that Andulasia was made up of a mixture of various races and cultures, and that consequently it was from these many cultures that Flamenco developed. Many Flamenco experts agree that in all probability the dance developed over the centuries among the gypsies, Jews and Muslims who were persecuted and exiled from Spain along with other outcasts.

Flamenco is a type of song and dance from Andulasia that has its roots in folk music and there are several specific styles of Gitano gypsy singing that are considered basic: siguiriya, tango, tona and solea.

The earliest forms of gypsy Flamenco were centred in the cities of Seville, Rhonda and Cadiz, which formed a geographical triangle with Jerez de la Frontera as its centre-point. A traditional Flamenco group consists of the dancer, the 'bailaor' or 'bailaora', the singer or 'cantaona' (male or female) and the guitarist, 'tocaor' or 'tocaora' (who was usually male). In Cadiz, then called Gades, the movements of the 'baile', meaning the dance, was more than likely influenced by Arabic dances. They are passionate, fiery, sinuous and lively. In contrast, at the seaports near Cadiz, the siguiriya is performed in a solemn and dramatic fashion, epitomising the dancer's sadness about death and the heartbreak of their struggles to survive the terrible vendettas against them.

The authentic country style of gypsy Flamenco, the Juerga (which is a term roughly equivalent to the American word 'jam session'), existed centuries before Flamenco became commercialised and was danced only on wooden staging and only to the cante, songs sung mainly by men within the gypsy community or in the privacy of their homes. These are light, joyous songs, followed by emotional lyrics expressing sorrow and pain, known as cante jondo.

Later, this dance or Juerga was performed on the streets and in commercialised premises such as theatres. It is now a special event, a spontaneous fiesta, a social gathering of Flamenco enthusiasts who enjoy the songs, dancing and the opportunity to eat, drink and reminisce. The Juerga is a passionate dance with the emphasis on the upper torso and arms, centred on the cante at the start of the fiesta.

The Tona, the oldest form of Flamenco, was only ever sung and never accompanied by finger-clicking or castanets. Such types of accompaniment to the dance were only introduced in the cafés-cantante in the 1900s. The guitar that we associate with Flamenco was not introduced as a solo Flamenco instrument until the 20th century.

During the 1860s, the dance began to flourish in the cafés-cantante in Madrid, Malaga and Seville, where members of the public could enjoy food and drink and be entertained.

The commercialised Flamenco, the 'Baile Grande', the dance seen mainly by tourists, is more commonly performed by the 'bailaor' (male dancer). It is also, however, performed by the 'bailaora' (female dancer) wearing a fitted, full-length, brightly coloured polka-dot dress with several layers of frills on the sleeves, neckline and around the bottom of the dress which swirl out effectively as she dances. Holding her head up proudly with eyes downcast, the dancer moves her hips, upper torso, hands and arms in movements very similar to those used in the belly dance, expressing through the dance her happiness and love of life. The 'bailaora' also performs the zapeado, a precise rhythmic stamping of the heels and toes, originally only performed by men.

The 'bailaor' dances with fiery passion, parading his masculinity, sexuality, virility and strength as he haughtily moves around the stage. He holds his body rigid and back arched in the traditional manner of the Flamenco baile dancer as he performs a complex and powerful routine of zapeado. Flamenco dancers are usually accompanied by singing, the guitar, finger-clicking and sometimes the castanets.

Cante, the authentic Flamenco singing, is without a doubt the most important aspect of Flamenco, from which dance and musical accompaniment take their direction.

It is probable that the 'Baile Grande' was in part a

combination of dances introduced by gypsies who had travelled from India and North Africa and settled in Spain. This greatly influenced the style of dances performed by the Arabs, who had seized and occupied Andulasia around 711 CE.

The Ghawazee Dancers of Egypt

The Ghawazee are the infamous female dancers recounted in the tales of European travellers of the 19th century (to which we will return later), and are arguably the main wellspring of Egyptian dance or belly dance. Originally, the term Ghawazee was used to refer to dancers from both Cairo and the countryside but developed to mean only those dancers from the rural areas, who dance in the traditional sense, adding little from ballet or other modern dance moves to their repertoire or style. However, as in my experience modern day belly dancers perform more or less the same movements as the Ghawazee dancers, so the terms will be used interchangeably here, the only difference being that the movements of the Ghawazee are generally more defined and less lewd.

The survival of Middle Eastern dance and music can mostly be attributed to the gypsies, particularly those who settled in Turkey, Egypt, North Africa and Spain.

The Ghawazee gypsies of the Al-Nawara tribe were Romanies from the Iberian Peninusla. They tended to stay in one place until some higher authority moved them on. Originally, they may have travelled from Persia to Syria from Northern India, making their way up towards Spain and then Eastern Europe where they resided for many generations. Eventually they settled on the banks of the Nile and in Cairo.

'Ghawazee' stems from the Arabic 'Ghawa', meaning 'invaders of the heart' or 'thieves of the heart'. The Ghawazee have always preferred to keep to themselves and preserve their own culture, which is said to pre-date Islam. For generations they continued the tradition of performing in the streets of their local towns and villages to entertain the passers-by, trying to earn a living as their ancestors had done for many generations previously. Many Ghawazee remained settled along the lower regions of the Nile, earning their living by performing lewd dances to entertain and going about their business in the hot, dusty, bustling streets and marketplaces. Often they would perform in front of a house or a courtyard, as it was thought improper to invite the Ghawazee into one's home or into a respectable harem to entertain. They were, however, frequently invited to entertain in the open air on festive occasions such as a wedding, birth or circumcision, and on many occasions they were invited to entertain men in houses of ill repute.

Some of the European travellers who witnessed Ghawazee dancing in the early 19th century maintained it had very little elegance. Edward William Lane, for example, in *Manners and Customs of the Modern Egyptians* (1836), writes, 'Their dancing has little of elegance; its chief peculiarity being a very rapid vibrating motion of the hips, from side to side.' They commented that although the performances would begin decorously enough, as their movements became more energetic and vibrant in time to the rapid rhythmic beat of castanets, darabuka and tambourines, their movements became much more lascivious, indecent and their gestures suggestive.

As the Ghawazee women dancers undulated, rapidly pushing their hips from side to side and swaying the upper parts of their torso, they were able to keep their lower torso motionless and vice versa, movements that dancers can only perform once they have perfected the art of isolation. Some of these dancers were able to control almost every muscle in their bodies. This enabled them to perform extraordinary feats such as quivering their breasts one at a time or both together, rolling and fluttering their abdomens, rippling the muscles of their arms and quivering from head to toe in a continuous rippling motion.

As the rhythm of the music changed to a slower tempo, the mood and movements of the dancers would change. With snake-like movements of their arms and body they would sink slowly to their knees, then arch their backs until their heads and shoulders touched the ground. While in this position, they would continue to wave their arms as they rippled their bellies, swaying and quivering their bodies. Rising from their knees, they would move slowly, undulating the lower half of their bodies. Then, awakened by the quickening beat of the music, they would repeatedly thrust their pelvises to and fro in a lewd, provocative manner, followed by a rapid shake of the hips as they rapidly pushed them from side to side with a little stomp of the feet. (This is a movement described today as the 'hip shimmy push'.) Very few street dancers were able to execute these extremely skillful movements, however.

In 1833, pressure from Islamic fundamentalists, other religious orders and members of the local public forced the Egyptian government to implement a major clampdown on nightclubs in Egypt and primarily Cairo, which prohibited dancers from performing or fraternising with customers. However, the plain-clothed police working undercover were easily outwitted by the shrewdness of the dancers' pimps or bodyguards, whose warning of the impending raids gave them plenty of time to exit the stage. They would be replaced by others dancers, usually foreigners, whose style of dance, although similar to that of the Egyptian dances, was less lascivious.

On his travels through Egypt in the 1840s, the novelist Gustave Flaubert (1821-80) wrote to a friend, saying how disappointed he was at not seeing any dancing girls as they were in exile in Upper Egypt, and lamenting that good brothels in Cairo had ceased to exist. He was referring to the 1834 edict introduced by Mohammed Ali, Governor and later Viceroy of Egypt, that prohibited dancing by female performers in Cairo and the deporting of all known courtesans to three other cities: Esna, Aswan and Quena. This action temporarily led to the closure of brothels and rid the streets of dancers. Even so, the ban was unsuccessful and by 1860 street dancers and prostitutes were back in business. Eventually all known prostitutes were taxed. This edict was followed six years later by taxation of all male and female dancers, an act from which Mohammed Ali's government is said to have greatly profited.

Efforts by the authorities in Cairo to curb the activities of the dancers and prostitutes continued. The women were confined to certain areas along the Nile. Those who worked on the streets in the Ezbekiyya area of Cairo were the first to be licensed under the regulating trade of 1896. Further regulations were then implemented to control the transmission of venereal disease by subjecting all known prostitutes to regular medical checks.

It was not until Flaubert and other Europeans, such as Lady Mary Wortley Montagu, Edward William Lane, Carsten Niebuhr and Lady Lucie Gordon-Duff travelled to the Middle East and wrote accounts of their experiences that there was any documentation about the dancers of Egypt.

Baron Dominique Vivant Denon, diplomat, artist and author of, '*A Journey to Upper and Lower Egypt*', was assigned to Napoleon Bonaparte's expedition to Egypt in 1789, during the military operations of General Bonaparte in 1802. He conceded that the dancers he witnessed on first impression were bonny and graceful but also claimed they were a little boring. That was until they became highly intoxicated with vast amounts of liquor, which they consumed as though it were lemonade. Then their dancing became unrestrained, lascivious and grossly crude. He also related that a sheikh refused to allow the dancing girls to perform in front of the French. The eyes of these infidels would defile them. However, the superior strength of the army forced the sheikh to relinquish his objections (*A Trade Like Any Other*, Karin Van Nieukwerk, 1995).

At a celebration in Roseta known as 'The Feast of the Prophet', Denon was not in the least impressed by a dance he witnessed and which he described as abhorrent, as it was performed by men in an indecent and sexually suggestive manner.

It was rumoured that a French general who regarded the young Ghawazee dancing girls who persistently trailed around the soldiers' camps as loathsome, ordered four hundred of them to be beheaded and their remains tossed into the Nile (*Belly Dancing*, Wendy Buonaventura, 1983).

Edward William Lane, who sailed from England to Egypt in 1825, observed that, when performing, the Ghawazee wore a dress similar in style to that worn in public by middle class women of Egypt. Their outfit consisted of two skirts worn one on top of another. An ankle-length skirt was put on first, and a shorter one that reached down to just below the knees was worn on top. In preference to a long skirt, some dancers wore Turkish-style trousers that were placed around the hips and gathered in around the ankles. The chemise was usually made of transparent white muslin, with long sleeves very wide at the elbow. Over the chemise they wore a long, fitted jacket, usually made of red satin, which was sometimes patterned, in tiger-like stripes. Around their hips they wore one of two shawls, tied either to the front or to the side. This greatly emphasised the movements of their hips. As an alternative they sometimes wore a silver girdle around their waists with high bosses (raised ornaments) from which hung masses of silver mascots and lucky charms. Added to this was a profusion of silver and gold jewellery that enriched their dresses, and also enhanced and emphasised their movements as they jangled and glittered whilst they swayed and shimmied.

Lane was said to have been extremely impressed by the Ghawazee and thought them very handsome and comparatively well dressed. He also believed, after studying Egyptian tombs, that the dance of the Ghawazee may have derived from a dance that was originally performed by Ancient Egyptians at private functions accompanied by various instruments. These dancers were depicted entertaining and amusing guests in the times of the early pharaohs in a highly salacious manner, wearing nothing more than transparent dresses, or in a state of nudity.

The names of kings found inscribed on monuments suggested to Lane that such dancing had been common in Egypt for centuries and was likely to have been practised even before the exodus of the Israelites (*Manners and Customs of the Modern Egyptians*, Edward William Lane, 1836).

Charles G. Leland (1825-1903) noted that costumes of the Ghawazee differed from those described by Lane. The costumes he described were garments of black that covered the women from head to toe, interwoven with silver stripes and prettily braided hair. Leland observed a dancer who wore a garment adorned solely with an incredible quantity of gold coins in all sizes, which noisily jangled as she danced. Some dancers wore their hair braided and decorated in many ingenious ways, with gold coins, jewels and silk threads terminating with silver balls that fell down below their shoulders from beneath their curiously shaped caps, which glittered and twinkled as they moved.

Carsten Niebuhr (1733-1815) and his companions, when on their travels through Arabia in the early 1800s, first observed the dancers briefly quite by accident and were not overly impressed. Towards the end of his visit to Egypt, he decided to gratify his and his companions' curiosity and alleviate their disappointment at having to depart by paying some dancing girls to entertain them as they waited for their ship in Cairo. At that time the Nile was very low, enabling dancers and musicians to entertain along its banks. Niebuhr and his fellow passengers were initially not at all pleased by the entertainment. He wrote the following account:

'Their vocal and instrumental music we thought was horrible, and their persons appeared disgustingly ugly with their yellow-stained hands, spotted faces, absurd ornaments and their hair larded with pomatum, but by degrees we learned to endure them and for want of a better way to fancy some of them as pretty, imagine their voices agreeable, their movements graceful though indecent and their music not absolutely intolerable.' (From the notes of Carsten Niebuhr following his expedition to the Yemen in 1762.)

The only women that travellers to the Orient such as Flaubert, Niebuhr and Lane ever witnessed dancing were prostitutes and public performers. These people were never allowed near a respectable harem or household to entertain while foreigners were unlikely to ever be invited into private houses. Prostitution has always been associated with street dancers, but in fairness not all dancers bestowed their sexual favours for money.

In spite of being plagued by the activities of vast numbers of Ghawazee, Levantine, Jewish and Italian whores and street dancers, the locals, who scathingly described these people as being physically unattractive, ugly and a nuisance, tolerated them to a certain degree.

Although considered of ill repute, Ghawazee dancing women were hired for private parties that were in less respectable homes, and when dancing unveiled before the men, they might also be observed by the women from the windows of their apartments or harems. Usually during such entertainment, a friend of the host collected small sums of money, and it was the practice to engage the Ghawazee for a specific sum. At many of the parties, there was little decorum or self-restraint, as the dancing women mingled with the guests, drank intoxicating liquor to excess and prostituted themselves. A common custom on such occasions involved men wetting a small coin with their tongues and sticking it onto the dancer's cheeks, lips or chin as she descended to the floor into a backbend. By the 19th century, this custom of tipping became known as 'nukoot'. It is still an accepted tradition for belly dancer to receive money while performing from keen members of the audience, who usually enjoy the opportunity of stuffing the money inside the bra or hip-band of the dancer.

When entertaining men at private events the Ghawazee wore nothing more than a transparent garment, often discarded during their performance. Sometimes they wore nothing other than a very full skirt, called a 'tob' or the 'shinitiyan', a pair of very baggy trousers (*Manners and Customs of the Modern Egyptians*, Edward William Lane, 1836).

People of Cairo tried to persuade themselves that there was nothing improper in Ghawazees dancing. The fact that women, who were not supposed to expose themselves, performed the dancing, led men who were not Ghawazees to dance in public in the same manner. These dancers were mostly Khawals, highly effeminate (according to Edward William Lane) male Muslims and natives of Egypt, who were frequently employed to dance in preference to women at the time. Their dress mainly consisted of a tight vest, a girdle and a type of petticoat. Their hair grew long like women's hair and they imitated the women by applying kohl to their eyes and henna to their hands and feet. In the streets when they were not dancing they would often veil their faces like the women.

The beautiful Kutchuk Hanem, a Turkish Ghawazee, whose name in Turkish means 'little princess', was a famous courtesan from Luxor in Upper Egypt in the mid 19th Century who originally lived in Cairo. Because of the influence of certain people close to her, she was able to remain in Cairo together with a handful of other dancers. She was the chief girlfriend of Mohammed Ali's son, but after falling out with him was quickly deported to Esna where Flaubert saw her as recorded in his, *Travels in Egypt* (1850).

On Flaubert's first visit to see Kutchuk perform, he marvelled at her movements as she danced for him and was so impressed by her that he begged her to dance for him again later that same day. The dance she performed was 'The Dance of the Bee,' during which she shed articles of clothing one by one until she was completely naked, saying that it was a dance she did not like to do for anyone, not even him. It is not known from whence 'The Dance of the Bee' originated, but it has been suggested that it may originally have been a frenzied fertility dance of Persian origin. It has been suggested that the dance gained kudos as the original striptease, but this has never been substantiated. On Flaubert's second visit to Kutchuk, four other women were also present, whom he described as 'blue stocking'. This was a term he used for whores who provocatively danced for him for several hours with interludes for sexual dalliance. After Kutchuk had danced, although she was exhausted, the besotted Flaubert made love to her and wrote:

'She was cold, so I covered her with my fur pelisse and she fell asleep, her fingers in mine. As for me, I scarcely shut my eyes. My night was a long and infinitely intense reverie, which was why I stayed watching that beautiful woman sleep. She snored, her head against my arm. I had slipped my forefinger underneath her necklace. She awoke and for an hour she warmed herself besides the brazier before returning to bed to fall asleep again.' (*Travels in Egypt*, Gustave Flaubert, 1850.)

It was in Esna that an American journalist, G. W. Curtis (1842-1892) also saw Kutchuk Hanem dance. He described her as not being particularly graceful but wonderfully gymnastic. She would jerk her muscles in time to the beat of the music, quivering every limb with great intensity as she clashed together her castanets noisily in her upraised arms throughout her performance.

Other Ghawazee were not particularly impressed by Kutchuk Hanem's performances and were very quick to criticise her. One of her critics was a dancer by the name of Aziza of Aswan, who introduced herself to Maxime du Camp, an intimate travelling companion of Flaubert, asking him if she could dance for him later. She stated that she was a far better dancer than Kutchuk and had a body more supple than that of a snake. Flaubert described her as tall, slender, black and charming in profile. Her dancing was much more supple that that of Kutchuck, much wilder, savage and more abandoned, more reminiscent of the black African style of dancing than that of the Egyptian dancers, which was generally more formal.

As Aziza danced to the rhythmic beat of the darabuka drum, she was accompanied by the constant clash of the castanets she held between her fingers. Her face remained expressionless as she jerked and thrust her hips furiously, quivering and shaking her arms until they rippled from her shoulders down to her wrists in a continual motion, and moving her hips and feet faster and faster as the tempo of the beat increased. According to his companions, Flaubert was terrified when she did the neck slide (sliding the head from side to side) as it looked to him as though her head was about to be decapitated. (*Travels in Egypt*, Gustave Flaubert, 1850.)

He did not agree, however that Aziza of Aswa was a much better dancer than Kutchuk or more expert. This was because he was biased. He was besotted by Kutchuk, and wrote down every detail about her in his notes:

'Her large dark eyes and split nostrils, a tooth that was beginning to decay, the fleshy folds of her stomach and full-shaped breasts that were covered only by fine purple gauze. The blue tassel of her Tarboosh [headwear] which was spread out like a fan over her shoulders and her black, wavy, unruly hair which was braided and tied back.' (*Travels in Egypt,* Gustave Flaubert, 1850.)

Flaubert also wrote a colourful summary about some male dancers in Cairo who entertained him in the dining room of a hotel:

'We have seen some male dancers. Oh. Oh. Oh. As dancers imagine two rascals quite ugly, but charming in their corruption, in their obscene leering and the effeminacy of their movements, dressed as women with their eyes painted with antimony. For costume they have wide trousers and an embroidered jacket. The latter comes down the epigastrium or upper abdomen whereas the trousers are held up by an enormous cashmere girdle folded double several times, being only about the pubis, so that the entire stomach, the loins, and the beginning of the buttocks are naked, seen through a black gauze, held tightly against the skin by the upper and lower garments. This ripples on the hips like a dark transparent wave with every movement they make. The music is always the same and goes on for two hours without stopping. The flute is shrill, and the drumbeats throb in your chest, the singer dominates us all. The dancers advance and retreat, shaking the pelvis with a short convulsive movement. A quivering of the muscles is the only way to describe it; when the pelvis moves, the rest of the body is motionless; when the breasts shake, nothing else moves. In this manner they advance towards you, their arms extended rattling bass castanets, and their faces under rouge and sweat, remain more expressionless than statues. By that I mean they never smile. The effect is produced by the gravity of the face in contrast to the lascivious movements of the body. Sometimes they lie down flat like a woman ready to be fucked, then rise up with a movement of the loins similar to that of a tree swinging back into place after the wind has stopped.' (*Travels in Egypt,* Gustave Flaubert, 1850.)

Flaubert went on to say it was too beautiful to be exciting and doubted whether they would ever find the women to be as good entertainers as the men.

In an extract from her famous *Letters from Egypt,* written during the period 1862-1869, Lady Lucie Gordon-Duff wrote describing her encounters with dancing girls at Keneh:

'At first I thought the dancing girls were queer and dull. One girl was very handsome but cold and uninteresting. One who sang was also very pretty and engaging, a dear little thing: But the dancing was...more or less graceful, very wonderful gymnastic feats and no more. But the captain called out to one, Latifeh, an ugly clumsy looking wench to show... what she could do, and then it was revealed to me. The ugly girl started on her feet and became the Serpent of the Nile, the head, shoulders and arms eagerly bent forward, waist in, and haunches advanced on bent knees, the posture, a cobra ready about to spring.'

Lady Lucie Gordon-Duff also wrote of other encounters with dancers and, like other travellers, found them dull, uninteresting and ungraceful. She was, however, greatly impressed by their wonderful gymnastic feats, in particular those dancing girls who moved their breasts 'first one then the other by some extraordinary effort'. (*Letters from Egypt*, Lady Lucie Gordon Duff, 1862-1869.)

During the 19th century, the Sharia Wagh-el-Birk, commonly known as the Ezbekiyya area, was a very popular haunt for dancers and prostitutes in Cairo struggling to make a living. It was a district with a unique character, perpetually buzzing with life with its numerous arcades, cafés and shops run by Arab merchants. In the markets, rickety stalls were piled high with colourful fabrics, fruit and vegetables, and a profusion of spices that culminated in a combination of aromas and pungent smells that hung heavily in the hot, dry atmosphere.

But it was the Ezbekiyya Gardens that proved most fascinating to European visitors, who flocked to witness the notorious dancers and whores who performed there. Mohammed Ali had originally created the gardens for the benefit of local people and European visitors, but sadly they became rather neglected and subsequently uninteresting, consisting of little more than some struggling patches of grass, a few trees and a little bird life. They were surrounded by railings, which vendors took the opportunity of using as rent-free stalls from which they sold tarbrushes, jewellery, dried nuts, beans and fruits, spices, ornaments, coffee and postcards.

At that time, this area of Cairo throbbed with activity twenty-four hours a day. The crowded streets were lined with coffee shops and numerous shabby stores selling cheap wares. Watersellers dominated in their traditional bright-red outfits, with tall, wide-brimmed hats decorated with pom-poms and bells that tinkled to attract thirsty passers-by. They would stroll among the snake-charmers, chestnut-sellers and fortune-tellers (who were more often than not Nubian women), as did the countless beggars and cripples who mingled among the jostling crowds in the hope of getting money from foreign visitors.

Along the narrow streets, preoccupied Arabs sat on chairs on crowded pavements outside the bars and music halls. They would leisurely pass the time by smoking their hukkahs (hubble-bubble pipes) and cigarettes, drinking beer or coffee while chatting to friends. They were often totally uninterested or perhaps just a little amused by the unattractive dancers wriggling and gyrating their flabby rolls of flesh in an ungainly fashion in front of them to the monotonous beat of darabuka drums and the tuneless clash of cymbals. To add to the confusion, heavily laden carts, precariously stacked with merchandise ranging from carpets to aromatic spices drawn by camels and braying donkeys, would trundle noisily over the cobble stones alongside the clattering din of the trams, somewhat drowning out the tuneless blaring of the brass bands.

This region became commercialised in the late 1800s, when a complex of coffee-houses, restaurants, theatres and cafés-chantants were developed, which gave entertainers an opportunity to perform behind closed doors in preference to the streets and marketplaces.

As with previous attempts to contain performers, however, this had little effect on the dancers or night club owners, who continued to prosper under the patronage of wealthy locals, overseas visitors and British and Australian troops who were posted to Egypt during the First World War.

After the First World War a new era for entertainers emerged in the Middle East because it became acceptable to attend theatres, concert halls and nightclubs. This in turn bestowed a certain degree of respect on some entertainers but it was not until the 1920s that belly dancing started to become acceptable and popular throughout the West as well as in the Middle East, as the result of its promotion through film and eventually television. In fact, it was not until as late as the mid-1990s that belly dancing became completely acceptable, largely due to the growing tourist industry which has meant that travellers to countries such as Egypt and Turkey return home with new found enthusiasm for the belly dance styles they have witnessed whilst abroad.

Many famous Egyptian dancers such as Taheyya Karioka, Naima Akef and Samya Gamal starred in highly popular Egyptian films, early to mid 20th century. Some Egyptian artists travelled to Hollywood to appear in films such as 'Salome', 'Cleopatra' and 'Samson and Delilah'.

The Ghawazee still tend to keep apart from other people and marry within their own tribal culture. Today there are only a small number of Ghawazee dancers from Luxor in existence. Each group has their own particular style of dance, which they have inherited from their ancestors and have managed to keep alive until the present day.

One of the very few families that still dance, and perhaps the most famous, are the Bawat Mazin of Ghawazee – 'bawat' meaning daughters or girls. There are nine daughters, Khayuah being the most well-known dancer, who were their father's bread and butter until he died several years ago. The eldest three danced together mainly to entertain tourists until they achieved their main ambition, which was to marry well within their own culture. Khayuah told me that she was the last of the Mazin daughters still dancing. She said there were other Ghawazee who had learnt the art through her sisters, but she does not consider them genuine because they did not inherit the art in the traditional way, that is, from mother to daughter. It should be in the blood, she says. Today, rather than pass the art onto their children as their ancestors have done for so many generations, the Ghawazee now prefer them to have a proper education. Khayuah recently told me she is preparing for her wedding, and once she is married, will stop dancing as tradition requires. If a Ghawazee marries a musician, however, this does give her an opportunity to continue dancing professionally and earn a living by entertaining the tourists.

The Ghawazee were always associated with the 'Moulids,' which were celebrations of Muslim saints' anniversaries. At these festive carnivals, the Ghawazee would have been an essential part of the entertainment with their traditional songs and dances. The Moulids are now no longer celebrated by the Ghawazee, but they still perform around their local towns and villages, at weddings and private local celebrations.

Nessim, the male singer and dancer of the group, is an amazing elder character, full of life and energy, who started by hanging around the Moulids and local weddings watching the Ghawazee perform. He learnt their style of dancing and singing and now performs in front of a group of musicians while the dancers take a well-earned break. While dancing, he beats out the rhythm of the drums with his feet, shakes his shoulder and slides his head from side to side. During part of his energetic act, he balances a beer bottle upon his head, descends to the floor until lying on his stomach, shakes his body, then rolls over two or three times before ascending. His balance and agility are extraordinary, and usually the beer becomes his at the end of his performance.

A style of dance known as the Raks al Saif, that is still practised among the Ghawazee and was said to be a speciality act of Fahneda Mahzar, a respected Egyptian dancer (referred to in the review of Donna Carlton's *Looking for Little Egypt* featured in *The Crescent Moon*, 1995), involves a tray of lighted candles balanced upon a bottle that sits on the head of the dancer. You have to have a great deal of confidence and skill to prevent everything from toppling while dancing and rolling over from side to side on the floor.

These gypsy groups and their dances that have survived for

hundreds of years have virtually disappeared. Sadly, it would seem that another unique and ancient culture of music and dance will soon be lost forever.

There is a unique series of dance videos providing a compilation of old black and while film clips of Egypt's most famous dancers, available by mail order from Ramzy Music International Ltd (www.hossamramzy.com).

Fundamentalism and its Effect on the Dance

The origin of the Islamic religion, Islam, meaning 'Will of God', was based on the revelations of the Prophet Mohammed, born in Mecca 570 CE. He was the son of a poor merchant and married a wealthy widow for whom he worked. During one of his frequent visits to the mountains on the outskirts of Mecca to seek solace and meditate, he proclaimed he had seen a vision of the Archangel Gabriel during which he said he had received a message appointing him to be God's special messenger, and to spread the teaching of a new faith centred on the one and only true God, Allah. In spite of much hostility towards him, by the time he died in 632 CE, the whole of Western Arabia had become Muslim. In the year of his death, his father-in-law Abu Bakr (632-634 CE) became the first Muslim Caliph and the chief defender of the Islamic faith.

Several years after Mohammed's death, a compilation of his doctrines was collected and recorded in written form by some of his most faithful followers. As a result a book was produced that became known as the Koran.

Between 634 and 650 CE, Muslims, driven by religious enthusiasm, conquered and destroyed Palestine, Iraq, Persia, Syria, Mesopotamia, Egypt and North Africa. By 711 CE the warriors had reached North West Africa.

After North Africa was defeated, the indigenous people, the Berbers, also became Muslim. Led by Arab armies, they crossed into the Straits of Gibraltar and invaded Spain. Eventually they reached France but were defeated by the French in 732 CE. By 750 CE, the great period of Arab domination was over though Islam continued to spread. From the 11th century onwards, Islam reached India, Asia Minor and South Russia. Legend has it that warriors holding the sword in one hand and the Koran in the other spread the word of Islam. The Islamic religion has continued to flourish over the centuries and it is estimated that there are now at least eight hundred million Muslims around the world.

Islamic restrictions have had a profound effect on all entertainers in the Muslim world. The orthodox Caliphs were starkly opposed to any form of entertainment that evoked impure thoughts and behaviour. Even so, for many centuries there was a much more relaxed attitude towards singers, musicians and dancers than there is today.

Today in many regions of the Middle East, particularly in Egypt, restrictions are enforced on dancers by Islamic fundamentalists to prevent them from contravening Islamic laws. All flesh has to be covered, particularly bare bellies, which are regarded as an extremely vulgar part of the dancers' anatomy, and feet have to be kept close together so as to prevent any part of their legs showing. In the early 21st century, only affluent Arab businessmen and tourists can afford to patronise the elite nightclubs in Cairo where the most famous belly dancers perform. Strict Islamic laws of the 1800s still govern these clubs, and fraternisation of the dancers with members of the audience, together with the showing of any bare flesh or performing immodest movements are banned – which of course restricts tradi-tional belly dancing movements and costumes considerably. Every dancer has to register with the moral police, who enforce the strict codes by turning up unexpectedly to check that the dancers are abiding by the laws.

From the 1970s to the 1990s, as a result of the rise of Islamic fundamentalism, many clubs and restaurants in Cairo that previously featured belly dancing were set on fire and the lives of many of the local dancers were seriously threatened. They lived in fear of reprisals against them and their families. Many have given up performing or have moved to other countries where they can practice their art freely and without threat.

The prejudice and attacks on venues and performers have seriously jeopardised the future existence of the belly dance and local exponents of the art in its country of origin. In recent times, the American University of Cairo was banned from importing books on the subject and president Hosni Mubarak made the decision to ban the dance from being shown on television in a bid to diffuse further attacks from the fundamentalists such as the Muslim Brotherhood and other extremists.

Belly dancers from England, America, Russia and Northern Europe have been coming to Cairo for years, much to the annoyance of some of the native dancers. Many of these dancers have adopted a style of dance they perform to modern music, which is acceptable to westerners but not to Egyptians or exponents of the art who say they much prefer the traditional style of dance and music that has evolved over the centuries.

There are fears that belly dancing will not survive for much longer, unless the Egyptians have the courage to embrace and promote this ancient dance. It is sad to see the decline of the oldest, most fascinating and colourful dance in the world, a dance from which all other styles of dance have derived. Let us hope that attitudes change and that Egyptians will once more embrace a dance culture that has such enduring appeal and is so passionately revered in many regions around the world.

A different attitude applies to the dance in some Western nightclubs where no restrictions are enforced upon the dancers. In a bid to encourage customers to consume large amounts of alcohol to boost profits for club-owners, dancers are encouraged to perform seductively, display as much flesh as they dare, and fraternise with the customers. Fortunately this insalubrious approach to the dance is not acceptable to the majority of performers who appreciate and respect the belly dance as an art form.

The Almehs

During the 8-9th century reign of Haroun Al Rashid called 'Al-Rashid The Upright' (Multilingual Wikipedia Online Encyclopaedia, www.wikipedia.org, 2003) which lasted from 786-809 BCE, the Ghawazee dancers outnumbered the singers so extensively that it was decided to train more singers to a much higher standard than previously. These highly trained singers were known as 'A'l'meh', an Arabic word meaning 'learned women'. By the 19th century, the Almeh women were often confused with the Ghawazee, but unlike the latter they were highly respected as entertainers and remained veiled. They were frequently invited by wealthy families and the nobility to entertain inside the harems or within their homes, an honour and privilege never bestowed upon the Ghawazee.

The men did not have the privilege of seeing the Almehs when they entertained women, and had to be content with just listening to their singing.

The Almehs were invited to dance and sing their songs of love and joy and to perform at important events such as weddings, births and circumcisions. Their dancing was of a highly sexual nature for they were also teachers in the art of lovemaking. The messages relayed through their body movements and gestures were a means of instructing others in sexual matters.

During his travels in the 1787, Savery M. Savery, a French traveller, was the first to witness and report on large numbers of dancing girls in Egypt (*A Trade Like Any Other*, Karen van Nieuwerk, 1995). He commented that:

> 'They are called Almeh [servants]. A more painstaking education than other women has earned them this name. They formed a celebrated community within the country and in order to join, one had to have a beautiful voice, a good possession of the language, a knowledge of the rules of poetry and an ability to spontaneously compose and sing couplets adapted to the circumstances, and know all the songs by heart. Their memory was furnished with the most beautiful moals-mawwals, which is a type of Yemenic folkloric song, and the prettiest stories. There is no fete without them; no festival where they did not provide pretty ornamentation.' (*Lettres Sur L'Egypt*, Savery M. Savery 1787).

Charles G. Leland was not as generous, however. He went with a friend to an Arab café-chantant in the Esbekiyya Gardens where the Almehs sang from behind thin curtains to the accompaniment of musicians. He compared their singing to a group of old Irish women wailing at a wake with a strong infusion of caterwauling.

He also witnessed and wrote about a delightful performance by a young dancer from Girgeh in Upper Egypt:

> 'Placing a cup, symbolic of temptation on the ground, she danced around it in a style which was perfectly Spanish, turning her body and sinking low with great grace and

exquisite art. The cup appeared to exercise terrible fascination, but she was afraid to drain it. Five times she lay on the ground with her thirsty lips just dallying from the edge, and then rising, swept in dance and thrilled and shivered, and turned, and sank again. The sixth time she completed a circle and no longer able to resist, she approached the cup with throbs and pauses, and then without using her hand, lifted it from the ground with her lips alone, draining it as she rose, and the tragedy of the temptation being over, merrily danced about the room in quick step, with her head thrown back, holding the cup all the time in her mouth.' (Charles. G Leland, 1873.)

He then described another dance performed on the same evening by an older woman, who placed a vase on her head and danced for a long time, using a great variety of movements without letting it fall. A younger dancer who performed a similar dance then joined her (Charles G. Leland, 1873).

Traditionally, Egyptian women were rarely instructed in the art of song and dance, but they enjoyed themselves immensely when, on occasion, professional entertainment was hired to amuse them. The entertainers were never employed solely for the mere amusement of women on a regular basis, however, as that would have been considered indecorous among respectable families.

The men always entertained separately from their wives, usually in the lower apartments of the house. Their wives would entertain their friends and relatives in the upper levels of the apartments or in the harem, which generally overlooked the court. The elaborate wooden lattice work of the windows prevented the entertainers from being seen. They could, however, be distinctly heard by the male guests gathered below in the courtyard or in the apartment.

Monts des Ouled Nail

In contrast to the negative attitudes and stigma directed towards the Ghawazee dancers and prostitutes of Egypt, there has never been any disrespect or animosity directed towards the young courtesans of the mixed Berber tribe that inhabit the Monts des Ouled Nail, extending approximately from Biskra to Jelfa. This is a nomadic Berber tribe from Algeria, the members of which still live in camel-skin tents in the searing, hostile Sahara desert. From an early age, these young women are encouraged to leave the security of their tribal homes. They roam the Sahara between Morocco and Algiers, stopping off at cities, towns and oases bordering the desert to sing and dance and sell their bodies to the men, an occupation not considered at all dishonourable.

Being inhabitants of Marabout and descendants of a saint the Algerian Mohammedans accepted the profession of the Ouled Nail as a religious rite. The women have traditionally been trained from a very early age to follow their tribal custom of dance and prostitution, and, when rich, to leave the profession to return to their tribe when it is assumed that as a matter of course they will settle down and marry well. The more wealth they accumulate through their profession, the greater their chances are of marrying into respectability. Once married, they never revert back to their profession, but train the younger generation to follow in their footsteps in keeping their tribal tradition alive – a custom that continues amongst whose who practise their profession.

According to a tribal legend noted in a publication called 'Desert Winds' written in 1927 by a European traveller to Algiers known only as 'Hafsa,' who spent some time with the Ouled Nail, this way of life for the women originated after one chief of the tribe forgave his beautiful young wife for her indiscretions during his absence while he was away at the war. So the profession we call 'prostitution' became a respected way of life for the women.

The evening's entertainment would begin with the beat of a drum, the shrill plaintive wails of the flutes and the mournful falsetto singing, together with the chanting or hand clapping of the other dancers. In the moonlight and half-light of the lanterns scattered around the camp, the dancers would take turns to dance, moving their bodies in a slow, sensual, hypnotic manner, undulating their supple hips with arms outstretched or half-raised, showing little expression on their dark, sensual, tattooed faces as their eyes followed the graceful movements of their hands. Suddenly the music would become lively and the swaying of their hips sexually tantalising, suggestive and passionate.

It was not unknown for these courtesans to disrobe completely as they danced, to highlight the muscular dexterity and suppleness of their lissom bodies as they rocked and thrust their pelvises, rippled each breast in turn and undulated their bellies rhythmically. Sometimes a bright precious jewel was placed in their navel, which emphasised their abdominal and pelvic area as being the focal point of their dance. Nudity also enabled them to show off their proficient skills in the art of seduction and lovemaking. Dancing to bewitch and entice an audience of men willing to pay handsomely for sexual gratification was for these young women a way of life. Their graceful hand gestures and finger-snapping may have originally been ritualistic in origin and is reminiscent of the hand movements of the Tauregs, who flick their hands in different directions.

The Ouled Nail girls used to wear an abundance of gold jewellery and coins around their ankles and necks, up the length of their arms and on their fingers, together with very large looped gold earrings. Their dresses of soft black material, which were sometimes decorated with gold threads and made up of several layers, covered them from head to toe, and to complete the effect, around their waists they wore a large decorated belt or girdle. Beneath a black head-dress embellished in a profusion of ornaments and gold coins, their beautiful jet black hair, which they would grease and entwine with plaits of black wool, fell beneath their shoulders. Their hands and feet would be decorated with intricate henna patterns that served a dual purpose: to ward off evil and denote which tribe they belong to. The amount of gold indicated the girl's prosperity and personal fortune. The more gold they had, the more respect they earned as courtesans. Sometimes their success would promote a little envy and dissatisfaction among other members of the tribe and would also attract the attention of thieves, who robbed or even murdered the dancer for their gold.

After Algeria achieved independence from France in 1965, the Ouled Nail's tribal way of life was threatened and it was difficult for the dancing girls to practise their profession openly. In spite of many difficulties, however, they managed to preserve their ancient tradition and continued to ply their trade among the tourists, Arabs and French soldiers in rooms or cafés. The Ouled Nail tribes of the Sahara have not yet completely disappeared and some continue to combine dance and prostitution as a means of making a living in the tradition of their ancestors.

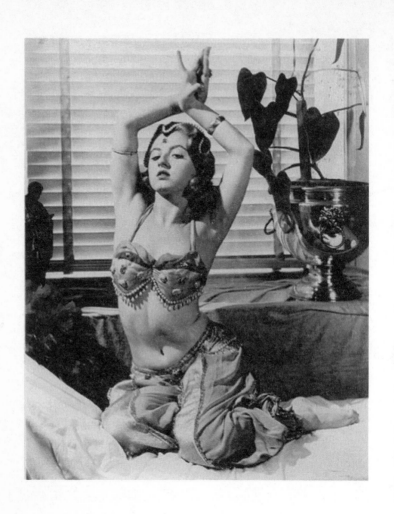

5

Belly Dance and the Harem

After the Roman Empire was split in the 3rd century BCE, Byzantium became the capital of the Eastern Empire. Renamed by the emperor Constantine as Constantinople in 324 BCE, it eventually became the capital of the Roman Empire, which spread westwards towards Spain over to the coast of North Africa, and northwards towards the River Danube. During the 10th Century BCE, however, it began to diminish, first under the onslaught of the Sejucks, a Turkish-speaking tribe, and then the Ottomans. The Ottoman State was one of many small Turkish states that emerged in Asia Minor during the breakdown of the Sejuck Turk's empire. However, the Ottomans went on to absorb the other states during a period of expansion during the 15th century that ended all local Turkish dynasties and established their status as a recognised European power. Within a century they progressed from being a nomadic people to the heirs of the most ancient surviving empire of Europe.

Following this initial period of expansion which saw their stronghold increase at the expense of the Byzantine Empire, Bulgaria, Serbia and the Balkan Peninsula, in 1453 CE led by Mehmet II or 'Mehmet the Conqueror' (1429-1481 CE) who was Ottoman Sultan from 1451-1481 CE, the Ottomans captured Constantinople and renamed it Istanbul. Superior military organisation enabled the Ottoman Empire to reach its zenith under the reign of Sulayman I or 'Sulayman the Magnificent' (1494-1566 CE), Ottoman Sultan from 1520-66 CE. His fleets dominated the Mediterranean. He was a great lawmaker and patron of the arts and architecture. At this time the Ottoman Empire covered an immense area that stretched from the Caucasian Mountains to the Persian Gulf and from the Danube.

During this period, the dance and music of the Turkish people successfully evolved side by side with dances from Damascus, Cairo and Baghdad. This resulted in some lasting changes to these art forms, which became the entertainment of the ruling elite. As a result, many Turkish influences in both classical and traditional folk music and dance have not only survived in Turkey to this day but are also evident in many areas of cultural life in the Middle East, North Africa and Central Asia.

The decay that followed Sulayman's death saw the clergy and the Janissaries (Christian conscripts to the militia renamed the corps of the Janissaries) gain power and exercise a corrupt and damaging influence. Through a series of treaties of capitulation from the 16th to the 18th centuries the Ottoman Empire lost its economic independence and the break-up of the state gained impetus with the Russo-Turkish Wars in the 18th century.

In 1821, Greece, which had been an integral part of the Ottoman Empire since 1460, rebelled against the Turks, who fought back and suppressed the revolt with ferocious barbarity. It was co-operation between the British and the Russians that secured the independence of the Greeks and led Turkey in 1829 to comply with the Treaty of Adrianople. Because of this treaty, in the 1830s the Egyptians were able to rid themselves of Turkish dominance.

Although Turkey was officially amongst the victors, the

country was left economically exhausted following the Crimean War. The Congress of Paris (1856) recognised the integrity and independence of the Ottoman Empire but this event marked the confirmation of the empire's dependency rather than of its rights as a European power. At the end of Mehmed VI's reign in 1922 the Ottoman dynasty formally ended and the 'sick man of Europe' was no longer.

After the First World War (1914-1918) and the collapse of the Ottoman Empire there were many dramatic changes in Turkey. Leading the country in its war of independence from 1919-1922 was the highly respected general Mustafa Kemal, who enabled a new Turkey to be established when the country was declared a secular republic with himself as president. He introduced social and political change, as well as western fashions, the emancipation of women, education reform and the Latin alphabet as a replacement for Arabic script. In 1935 Kemal took the name 'Ataturk' or 'Father of the Turks,' (*Cambridge Biographical Encyclopaedia*, ed. David Crystal, 1998).

The Harem

In Ancient Egypt the harem was simply the room in the house occupied by the unmarried women and could include the mother, the grandmother, the householder or even the mistress of the house as well as any female servants or slaves. However, since the practice of keeping a harem was most often associated with the sultans of the Ottoman Empire, who, according to the Koran, were allowed to keep as many as four wives, and who, according to Turkish law, could also keep any number of male slaves, eunuchs, female slaves and concubines; the term conjures up images somewhat less innocent than the simple living arrangement of the Ancient Egyptians.

The concept of having large numbers of women locked up for the convenience of a sultan, though made famous by the Ottomans, in fact came to them from the Byzantines. Before coming to Anatolia, Turks did not have harems but once Istanbul had been captured and the construction of the city's famous Topkapi Palace was underway, the introduction of the harem was initiated as the sultan built a harem parallel to Topkapi, as his family's living quarters. It was not only in Turkey that the practice of keeping a harem was widespread. In Ancient Egypt for example, there were private quarters within wealthier homes, particularly within royal residencies, where women only lived. In Egypt, as in other Mediterranean societies, the honour of men and the family rested upon the sexual purity of women and often the keeping of a harem was as much to do with protecting this purity as with flouting wealth or using the harem as a social convention indicating economic standing.

Although the Ancient Egyptian word for harem was 'ipet' or 'per-khemret', meaning private rooms or apartments, the word 'harem' stems from the Arabic 'harim', meaning unlawful or forbidden. The term was originally used to refer to certain areas within a Muslim city considered holy or sacred where only the faithful may enter and where certain activities were prohibited. So 'harem' was used to refer to a section of a Muslim house occupied only by women, an inner sanctum. It is also used to refer to the group of women occupying these rooms. The Turks modified the word harem by adding 'lik'. Thus 'haramlik' in Turkish is the correct word for the quarters inside the house allocated to the wife, children and servants.

Within the harem would exist a hierarchy of favourites, 'Royal Wife' being the highest position followed by a number of 'favourites'. Within Turkish harems there were usually four different classes, namely the odalisques or servant girls; the gedliki, who were the sultan's personal servants and usually numbered twelve; ikbal or gozde, who were favourites said to have affairs with the sultan; and the kadin or haseki sultan, who were the wives giving children to the sultan. When the haseki sultan's son ascended to the throne she was promoted to valide sultan or 'queen mother' and became the most important female of the harem. The sultan's daughters were next, followed by the wives who had given birth to children for the sultan and whose rank depended on the order in which their sons had been born.

The status of the women and the privileges accorded them was also influenced by their relationship with the sultan, this being largely dependent on the women's beauty, charm and talent. The women of the harem were known as 'the adorned ones' and as their existence consisted of pleasing their master, they were expected to sing, play instruments such as the lute, lyre and harp as well as being able to dance.

The influence of the Harem women upon affairs of the court would fluctuate according to the character of the sultan ruling at the time and depending on his relationships with the women of the harem but the women often exerted considerable power over the sultan's political decisions. From 1541-1687 the 'favourite wives' were influential to such an extent that this period became known as the 'Reign of Women'. The women of the harem exerted influence to a greater or lesser degree, first with the Sultan Murad, then with Bayezid, Muhammed, 'Selim the Grim' (ruling from 1512-1520 BCE) and 'Sulayman the Magnificent' (1520-1566 BCE). Some historians believe the influence of the women was the cause of the beginning of the Ottoman decline although not the ultimate reason for its downfall. In fact, the eventual decay of the empire was the result of the actions of a long line of incompetent sultans together with reasons mentioned earlier in this chapter.

In 1462 CE and almost a decade after his conquest of

Constantinople, Mehmet II 'the conqueror' (1429-1481 CE) decreed that a new municipality be constructed that he named Istanbul. This was a development of magnificent and ostentatious buildings surrounded by walls overlooking the intersection of the Bospherous and Marmara Sea and the Golden Horn, the curved inlet of the Bospherous that became the Arcropolis of Ancient Byzantium.

The Topkapi State Palace was built from 1466-1478 CE, several years before the demise of Mehmet the Conqueror, and was itself a city consisting of many fountains and beautiful gardens full of scented flowers, plants and trees, colourful exotic birds, and a variety of animals. It had exquisitely decorated pavillions, libraries, marbled halls, a palace school, bath houses and residences, and was built on the Seraglio Point overlooking both the Marmara and Bosphorus.

The palace also contained several mosques, a military school, ten huge kitchens and flour mills, two bakeries and numerous storerooms. Apartments were divided into rooms for the harem, concubines, eunuchs, odalisques or female servants (from the Turkish word 'odaliq' meaning 'chamber maid') and the sultan's numerous wives.

Gradually the compound was split into four courtyards by four interior walls and the final form of the palace covered 7000 km^2 enclosed with a fortified wall stretching 1400 metres in length. The Grand Seraglio was the Royal Palace, the seat of imperial power which accommodated hundreds and thousands of employees assigned to work in the sultan's administrative and personal service. However, the sultan's private quarters, his harem, were separate from the rest of the palace. It was not until 1541 CE that it was moved to the Seraglio with the advent of Sultana Roxelena.

In spite of opulent excesses, the activities of the palace appeared to attract little interest, mainly because idle curiosity was entirely centred on the secret and mysterious intrigues of life inside the harem. No visitors, not even foreign ambassadors, were allowed to enter this very private and secret domain. What little information did filter into the world outside was usually unreliable, consisting of tales told by eunuchs or odalisques.

Topkapi Palace in Istanbul, known to the Turks as Top Kapi Saray, became known in the West as the 'Seraglio', the summer palace or sublime port. 'Seraglio' is an Italian adaptation of the Persian word 'Serraclio,' meaning a cage for wild animals, and was used because of its similarity to the Persian words 'saray' that originally meant a palace or building. The word 'sarai' was primarily used by the Tartars but became 'serail' and 'seraglio' in the language of the Levantine Franks before being adapted to eventually mean the 'The Royal Palace of Ancient Acropolis up on the hill.' The headland on which Topkapi stands became known as the Seraglio Point and is still known as that today. Over the years, tourists in Istanbul wishing to visit the Seraglio asked to be taken to the Topkapi, a term that now carries the same meaning

Over a period of four hundred years lasting from about 1540 to the early 1900s, the sultans of the Ottoman dynasty kept their women in isolation, completely hidden from the outside world. In the Topkapi alone, thousands of women lived and died within the confines of the harem, knowing only each other and some of the eunuchs.

Slavery was a successful commercial enterprise in and around the Middle East 4000 years ago. Women who entered the harem as slaves were bought in the open slave market. Their ages ranged from as young as twelve to women in their fifties. They were often abducted from or sold by their destitute parents.

Many of these unfortunate women were seized from the Abkhasian and the Caucasian regions. Later, they were bought using peaceful means. Some were even sent as gifts from Egypt to the Pashas.

Eunuchs were male salves or prisoners who became the property of their conqueror. White eunuchs, like the women, were available from many conquered regions, including Georgia, Circassia and Armenia, but they proved to be rather feeble in comparison to the black males who were less delicate and much cheaper.

Although white and black eunuchs were employed in the Seraglio, all communication between them was strictly forbidden. As N. M. Penzer wrote in *The Harem* (1936), 'No white eunuchs are allowed to visit their back brethren in any circumstances whatsoever. Each had his own distinct duties.' White eunuchs were responsible for overseeing the court pages and their numerous activities and provided a personal service to the sultan as members of the royal household. Although white eunuchs were originally preferred, increasingly black eunuchs were more frequently employed to oversee the harem as it was thought they would be less attractive to the women and any children born to the women of the harem could be more easily identified as not of the master's seed.

Kapi Agha was the chief white eunuch employed at the Royal Palace and had many privileges. Primarily, he was allowed to speak to the sultan alone in his private quarters, act as his personal confidant and oversee any confidential matters addressed to him. He was privy to the sultan's most intimate secrets.

He was acting head of the palace school and of the infirmary, Gatekeeper in Chief, Inspector of Mosques and Masters of Ceremonies. Kapi Agha reigned supreme until many of his privileges and authority were transferred to his black rival the Kisla Aghar or chief black eunuch, by Sultan Murad III in 1591. The power of the white eunuchs had previously been greater than that of the blacks but because of corruption, mistrust and embezzlement, their power declined and they met their downfall. Their authority was gradually transferred to the black eunuchs.

This loss was of great concern to Kapi Agha as he had much to lose including his position as the women's chief, together with many other authoritative and lucrative posts.

Kisla Agha assumed the same privileges and prestigious responsibilities as Kapi Agha and was honoured with many distinguished titles. His many duties included officiating at royal ceremonial events, providing women for the harem, protecting and escorting women and screening any woman who requested an audience with the sultan. He had the privilege of liaising between the sultan and the valide sultana, the sultan's mother, and acted as their intermediary. He was described as, 'The most illustrious of the officers...worthy of the confidence of monarchs and of sovereigns...The door to his bedroom was on the south side of the palace opposite the sultan's,' (*The Harem*, N. M Penzer, 1936).

The chief black eunuch exercised immense political powers in court and his rank was as high as that of the Grand Vizier, whose role it was to oversee the running of the government on a day-to-day basis and act as prime minister to the sultan. He became a very powerful and feared man and the most bribed official in the entire Ottoman Empire. Described as corrupt, crude and ignorant, the chief black eunuch is credited with playing a significant role in its decline and fall.

Hundreds of eunuchs were sent to the Seraglio to act as guardians to the sultanas (who were the many 'wives' of the sultans), concubines and odalisques. They were also acquired to carry out business transactions and were trusted to receive and deliver messages between the sultan and his sultanas, but they were not allowed to leave the Seraglio without the permission of the sultana.

Within the Seraglio, rules and regulations had to be strictly observed. It was the valide sultana who presided over the harem. Her position of power was very great. She demanded obedience from every member of the harem and refused an audience with any of the sultan's official wives unless an appointment had been made.

Once the slaves had passed through Topkapi Palace's 'Gates of Felicity', which were symbolic of their entering into the sultan's harem for life, there was no turning back. However, for many women, peasant girls in particular, this was less of a 'life-sentence' and rather a window of opportunity as the privileges afforded the women of the harem as they moved up within the harem's ranks were great. For example, one of Selim III's 'favourites', the bas kadin Nurbanu, had an entourage of no less than one hundred and fifty handmaids.

Very few first hand accounts ever became known about the lives of the women who lived within the confines of the harem until their deaths. However, from the reports that have emerged it seems that for most inhabitants life within the walls of the harem was more than likely to have been extremely dull. (This is except for those astute enough to understand that where they lived afforded the opportunity to acquire luxury and riches once they had won the sultan's favour.)

Constant bickering and jealousy was rife and boredom was relieved by poetry readings, dancing and playing instruments like the lyre, harp, lute and the sistra. The harem women also had the occasional trip on the Bospherous. They made up shadow-shows that were full of obscenities but hugely popular and had sexual liaisons with eunuchs and between themselves. There was also evidence that the occult was practised within the harem, including exorcisms, fortune telling and other superstitious practices intended to predict the future.

Dancers were trained within the confines of the harem. Occasionally pantomime artists and some passing public dancers and singers including Almehs and Bayaderes or 'Natchees' or 'Maikos' (professional dancers whose moves were focused on the waist upwards), often with breasts exposed, were brought in from the outside world as a distraction and accepted with great enthusiasm and joviality. The nature of their dancing was far from modest. N. M. Penzer wrote that the dancing he had witnessed in the Topkapi was extremely lascivious, lewd and erotic (*The Harem*, N. M Penzer, 1936).

During the reign of Selim III, 1789-1809 CE, a group of musicians and a French teacher escorted by black eunuchs were granted permission to enter the buildings surrounding the harem to give dancing lessons to women selected to perform in a show. Those chosen were usually young girls whose union with Islam had not yet been consolidated.

For his own personal pleasure and entertainment the sultan sometimes admitted entire members of his harem into the Hunkar Sofasi, the throne room or hall of the sultan which was a long, elegant and rectangular room with a raised platform overhanging a balcony at one end. When seated on his throne, the sultan was a magnificent sight dressed in scarlet robes trimmed with sable together with a turban with a white egret (plume) secured with a cluster of rubies and emeralds and with a bejewelled waterpipe at his side. He would be surrounded by his most ravishing favourites known as the kadins and the valide sultana reclining on an array of colourful luxurious embroidered cushions. Tradition allowed only four prinicipal kadins, who were equivalent in rank to that of a legal wife, but an unlimited number of concubines. The sultan would also be entertained by the chengis dancing girls who whirled, swayed and undulated suggestively in groups before their king, each vying for his undivided attention. (He would often also be entertained by effeminate male dancers dressed as females). Odalisques were not allowed to be seen sitting in the presence of the sultan but were able to witness events at some distance whilst unobtrusively lolling against the walls of the great hall.

The beauty of the harem women on such occasions was a dazzling and spectacular sight. Each would be dressed in colourful garments of silk and satin, velvet and muslin, embellished in jewels, precious stones and ornaments of every description.

The principle women of the harem would be extravagantly attired from head to toe in rich brocades, cashmere and velvets, fine silks and satins and robes, lined with either sable or ermine. Their exquisite and dazzling outfits would be adorned with an abundance of jewellery made up of diamonds, rubies, emeralds and pearls that flashed and sparkled as they moved.

All the women wore chemises and trousers of fine linen or muslin that would modestly cover their legs, shoes of white kid leather embroidered with gold and little caps made of velvet, silver or gold fabric. Some would dress their long hair, divide it into tresses and braid it with pearls or ribbons, flowers, feathers or a cluster of jewels.

In 1717, Lady Mary Wortley Montagu wrote a number of letters of literary worth during her husband's appointment as Ambassador Extraordinary to the Court of Turkey. Specifically, in a letter she wrote to her sister dated April 1st 1717, she described one costume she wore as follows:

'The first piece of my dress is a pair of drawers, very full, that reach to my shoes and conceal your legs more than your petticoats. They are of thin rose damask brocaded with silver flowers. My shoes are of white kid leather embroidered with gold. Over this hangs my smock of fine white silk gauze, edged with embroidery. This smock has long sleeves, hanging half way down the arm and is closed at the neck with a diamond button; but the shape and colour of the bosom very well to be distinguished through it. The antery is a waistcoat made close to fit my shape, of white and gold damask with a gold fringe, and very long sleeves falling back and with diamond or pearl buttons.

My caftan, made of the same stuff as my drawers, is a robe exactly fitted to my shape and reaching to my feet, with very long straight falling sleeves. Over this is the girdle of about four fingers broad which all that can afford have entirely of diamonds or other precious stones; those who will not manage that expense have it exquisitely embroidered on satin but it must be fastened before with a clasp of diamond. The curdee is a loose robe they throw off or put on according to the weather, being of rich brocade (mine is green and gold) and lined either with ermines or sables. The head-dress is composed of a cap, called a talpock, which is in winter a fine velvet embroidered with pearls and diamonds and in summer of light shining silver stuff. This is fixed on the one side of the head, the hair is laid flat; and here at liberty the girls show their fancys; some putting flowers, others, a plume of heron's feathers and in short what they please; but the most general fashion is a large bouquet of jewels, made like natural flowers; that is, the bud of pearl; the rose of different coloured rubies; the jessamines of diamonds, the jonquils of topazes etc. The hair hangs at its full length behind, divided into tresses braided with pearl or ribbon, which is always in great quantity.'

The gomlek was a long, loose shirt or chemise worn down to the knees; made from either a mixture of wool or cotton or silk gauze which was usually white but also dyed in yellow, blue and red, with loose wide sleeves edged with lace or satin. Until the fashion was modified it was usually left open down to the waist exposing the breasts.

The outer trousers, salvar or chalwar, were very widely cut, drawn in at the waist, looped up below the knees and fell in folds around the ankles. The long drawers Lady Montagu wore were called dyslik or dislik and were very widely cut, drawn around the waist and tied at the knees. The entari, worn inside the harem, was a waistcoat fitted like a corset.

The entari was wide open in front and when the gomlek was in fashion the bosom remained entirely exposed. It was fastened at the waist by pearl or diamond buttons set close together and like a waistcoat or corset fitted tightly. The sleeves were fitted from the shoulder down to the elbow and hung down nearly to the ground exposing the sleeve of the gomlek from the elbow to the wrist.

The little hats described by Lady Montagu were head-dresses worn inside the harem. Yasmaks or yashmaks were veils exclusive to Istanbul and always worn by women when outside the home. The veil consisted of two pieces of very fine muslin. The first piece was placed across the bridge of the nose, fell over the mouth and chin down to the bosom, and was fastened at the nape of the neck. The second piece was placed over the head and brought down over the front above the eyebrows. The rest hung down behind either pinned to the other half of the yashmak or tucked into the outer robe. The only area of the body exposed was the eyes.

When strolling outdoors around the gardens, the women would wear shoes or slipper-like boots called cedik that curled up at the toes and were usually made of yellow Moroccan leather.

Opium was originally used as a medicine but it became very popular among the women who began using it for pleasure and as a means for forgetting their isolation, relieving their anxieties and sexual frustrations.

Much of the dancing performed in the confines of the harem was extremely suggestive as dancing was one of the few avenues through which the women were able to relieve their sexual frustration, get some physical exercise and amuse one another.

As sexual activity was rife to a certain extent harems became almost like brothels. Lesbianism was commonplace, and when dancing for one another, one of the women would assume the role of a male and imitate the sex act by performing the dance movements in a very indecent and lewd manner in pursuit of sexual satisfaction.

All eunuchs were deprived of their full sexual capabilities, but those who had been castrated at puberty and had lost only one testicle could still get an erection. They would have passionate affairs in secret with the women they guarded. Islam forbade castration and it is believed that the operation was usually performed outside Istanbul.

The women preferred eunuchs in preference to other men probably because they were far less likely to become pregnant. Eunuchs were said to be very skilled lovers, particularly in the art of oral sex, and quite unselfish in their sexual pursuits. This made them very popular with the women of the harem. Marriage between eunuchs and odalisques in the Seraglio was not an uncommon event but once married they had to live outside the harem.

Sexual liaisons could result in serious punishment or even death. After hearing of a concubine's sexual encounter with a eunuch, Sultan Ibrahim 'the mad' (1616-1648 CE) went into a fit of rage and demanded that over 250 harem women be tied in sacks, weighted down with stones and tossed into the Bospherous. Only one survived to tell the tale, having managed to escape from the sack, probably because it had not been tied securely. She floated to the surface where she was allegedly picked up by a French boat and taken to Paris.

Many unfortunate women were severely punished and more often than not ended up at the bottom of the Bospherous or Marmara Sea for their indiscretions, petty or serious crimes that usually came to the attention of the chief eunuch through gossip or informants.

During the reign of Muhmud II (1808-1839) his mother, Amie de Rivery, helped to relax the strict social structures within the harem to give the women more freedom. Although heavily guarded by eunuchs, they were able to take kayaks for pleasure trips down the Bospherous and picnic in the meadows while being entertained by dancing bears, acrobats, dancers and musicians. They would also watch puppet shows which were very popular.

Turkish Dance

Dance has always played an important role in the lives of the Turkish people, in religious ceremonies, pageantry and within their own communities for enjoyment or to celebrate a wedding or circumcision.

During the occupation of Turkey from 1520 to 1924 CE by the Ottoman Turks, the music made by musicians, singers and dancers successfully evolved side by side with the music of the neighbouring countries of Egypt, Iraq and Syria. Consequently, Turkish influences are still present in many areas of cultural life in North Africa and Central Asia and this is clearly evident in the fields of music and dance. Turkey is remarkably rich in both folk music and dance styles, particularly evident in Central Anatolia, the heartland of Turkish culture and the Black Sea coast.

Turkish gypsies, known as the Zingarri, exerted a great deal of influence on dance and music forms over the centuries. During the Ottoman Period, they become organised and formed entertainment guilds. They were employed to dance in the courts of Edirne, formerly Adrianople, in Istanbul and Bursa, an industrial town in North West Turkey and the capital of the Ottoman Empire from 1326 to 1413 CE.

The improvised styles of dance that originated from the

Turkish gypsies and that are still performed today, are known as the 'Ciftetelli'. This literally means 'two strings' and is a Turkish drum rhythm in 8/4 line tempo that also refers to an improvised musical section by a solo instrument carrying the melody, that is layered over the top of that pulsing rhythm. The most important musical styles used in the Ciftetelli are the composed instrumental forms Semai and Pesrev and the improvised Karsilama and Dolab, which is a very fast rhythm of 9/8 and which means 'face to face'. The structured progression of melodic modes function as a prelude to the dancers' entrance and may be played in turn by individual instruments such as the violin, oud and kanoon – an instrument not unlike the zither.

Metin And, an expert on Turkish folk dance (www.zehara.co.uk), affirms that there are notable similarities between Turkish folk dances and the dances of the Balkans, that is, Romania, Serbia and Greece. Metin places the dances of Turkey into three separate categories: folk dances, religious dances (from which Sufi dances emerged), and exhibition dances. He believes that Turkish dance developed on two different levels. Hundreds of peasant folk dances were danced for pleasure in remote villages, which probably helped to preserve them. Then there were the more formal and complicated dances of the city dwellers in Istanbul that developed under the influence of the court at the time of the Ottoman Empire.

There are as many as fifty eyewitness accounts of dancers in Turkey who entertained in the houses of the wealthy. The women who danced were described as being extremely beautiful and magnificently dressed, attended by their slaves whose role was to take great care of their mistresses' clothing. Once the ladies had been seated and served refreshments, the most distinguished 'Cengi' (Turkish dancer) of the company arose to dance for just a few minutes, then adjourned to her apartment in which her slave was waiting, to assist her in changing her dress.

Meanwhile other dancers would perform separately and would then in turn depart to change their dresses. This sequence would be repeated many times during the course of an evening. Each costume was more decorative and elaborate than the previous, heavily embroidered in gold and silver. Only the same head-dresses and bracelets, which were ornamented in a variety of sparkling jewels, were retained by the dancers while performing throughout the evening and in spite of other costume changes.

Lady Mary Wortley Montagu was the first European traveller to include in her correspondence comments about dancers in Turkey that she witnessed in 1717. She describes the experience as follows:

> 'She made them a sign to play and dance. Four of them immediately began to play some soft airs on instruments between a lute and guitar, which they accompanied with their voices while the others danced by turns. This dance was very different from what I had seen before. Nothing could be so artful or more suited to raising certain ideas, the tunes so soft, the motions so languishing, accompanied with pauses and dying eyes, [the dancers] half falling back then recovering themselves in so artful a manner that I am positive the coldest and most rigid prude on earth could not have looked upon them without thinking of something not to be spoke of.' (*The Complete Letters of Montagu,* Lady Mary Wortley Montagu, 1917.)

Little Egypt

In the 19th century, very little was known in the West about belly dance. People first experienced the dance in the USA when it was brought to the Midway Plaisance, a strip of land which connected Jackson Park to Washington, where the Chicago World Fair was staged in 1893.

The World Fair incorporated a fantasy world which gave straight-laced Americans a glimpse of the exotic east. There were kiosks and bazaars; a typical Kabyle house showing the spatial arrangement of the homes of the Kabyle people (Berbers of Algiers and Tunisia); a Bedouin camp; village exhibits of Turkey and Algeria; a replica of a mosque and a replica of the Luxor Temple as well as a great amusement park that had a large Ferris wheel and many other attractions. Organisers of the World Fair 1893 saw it as an opportunity to introduce historical, cultural and educational exhibits to both American and foreign visitors.

'Cairo Street' or simply 'The Street' as it became known, was an outstanding spectacular exhibit that enraptured the public and proved to be the most popular part of the fair. 'The Street' featured a theatre where snake charmers and dancers performed. There were daily festivals and processions, sometimes to celebrate a Moulid (Arab celebration of saint's day) or maybe a wedding. Donkey and camel rides were great novelties and were considered immense fun. There were street vendors, fortune-tellers, young acrobats, musicians playing their instruments with strange rhythms and singers filling the air with wailing and melodious songs.

Orientals who strolled the street and occupied the booths in their resplendent national costumes included people from the Levant, Greeks, Sudanese, Arabs and Turks, Copts, Muslims, Jews, Armenians and Nubians. The combined effect of the people and the attractions gave the Americans a taste of Eastern exotica at this extraordinary historic pageant.

The 'Cairo Street' theatre dancers were said to have been given many names, the most popular being simply the 'Dancing Girls'. Their dances were called many different names, such as 'Danse du Ventre', 'muscle dance', 'contortion dance', 'nautch dance', 'oriental posture dance' 'the ballyhoo' and the 'hoochy coochy,' which was eventually referred to as the 'coochie dance'.

Fahreda Mahzar, a Syrian dancer who claims to have danced at the fair, is thought by some to have been the infamous dancer known as 'Little Egypt'. Wendy Bounaventura, for instance, asserts that Fareda Mahzar danced at the Chicago World Fair under this name (*Serpent of the Nile*, Wendy Bounaventura, 1994). Others claim to the contrary, for example, Donna Cartlon in her book *Looking for Little Egypt (1995)*, says the dancer who first called herself 'Little Egypt' was in fact a woman named Ashea Wabe.

We do not know much about Little Egypt, except that she was a strong, rebellious character, born in Damascus. She moved to and settled in Cairo where she acquired her professional skills in oriental dance. She emigrated to America in her mid-teens, and began to work as a professional dancer. After her marriage in 1905 to Gus Spyropolous, a restaurateur, she more or less retired from dancing. Her final performance was at the Centre of Progress at the later 1933-4 World Fair in Chicago. She died in Chicago in 1937.

The Syrian dancers were a huge success and attracted large crowds although the dances themselves shocked American audiences. In a review of the fair, it was admitted that the dancers were an instant success and that their gyrations and contortions had attracted enormous crowds. The dancers, however, were described as vulgar, unattractive and lacking in grace.

Sol Bloom, an impresario who was responsible for the installation of the exhibits and who looked after the payment of the performers, was delighted, because he made huge profits. His opinion of the dancers was therefore much more flattering.

Although popular with the public, who admired their

muscle control, the Ghawazee dancers rarely received praise at the fair. As in Egypt, their appearance was described as loathsome and their gyrations lewd. Both secular and religious groups disliked them.

Little attention was paid to the Turkish or Algerian dancers. Nevertheless, the handkerchief dance presented in the Algerian Village theatre was said to be 'most pleasing'. Throughout Maghreb (Algeria, Tunisia and Morocco) professional dancers included the handkerchief dance in their repertoire. When performing the pantomimic handkerchief dance, the dancer told a tale through her varied gestures and postures.

Although travellers from the early 1800s had used the term 'belly dance', it was claimed that Sol Bloom coined the phrase belly dance from the French phrase, 'Danse du Ventre,' said to be the name of a particular dance of the Ouled Nail of Algiers.

There is little doubt that Little Egypt's success encouraged other Egyptian dancers to ply their trade in the West and especially in the USA. This led to many dancers being employed to entertain at other World Trade Fairs, particularly in Paris, London and Chicago, to help promote the expanding industrial revolution. In turn, the influx of dancers from Egypt to the United States prompted western dancers to try their luck in Egypt. It is possible that they were influenced by the style of dance performed by the Egyptians and that the Egyptians were also influenced by the western style of dance. In any event, there eventually resulted a combination of the two forms of dance, from which today's modern form of the belly dance is likely to have evolved.

The Dance of the Seven Veils

In 1910 in Chicago, a dancer named Mary Garden, prima donna of the Chicago Opera Company (1874-1967), performed at the company production of 'Pelleas et Melisande,' stunning her audience and causing an outrage with her 'Dance of the Seven Veils'. The Chicago Chief of Police, Leyroy T. Stenard, found Gardener's show disgusting. He said he could find no artistic merit to her programme and compared her dance to 'a cat wallowing in a bed of catnip'. Because of this reaction, the management ended the show's run to avoid an official closing. Unperturbed, Mary Garden then travelled to Milwaukee to perform her dance again, only this time it was received with disinterest and very little comment.

Following in the footsteps of Mary Garden, other exotic dancers and striptease artists began to emerge during the earlier part of the 20th century, who combined the use of a veil with some movements of the belly dance. Many believe that the use of the veil originated with belly dancers in the Middle East, but it is likely that exotic American entertainers at least popularised the use of the veil even if they did not introduce it.

The 'Dance of the Seven Veils' is said to symbolise the seven gates through which the Asiatic goddess of love, Ishtar, passed through on her journey to the underworld. Ishtar was also the goddess of the planet Venus and worshipped as the queen of beauty and love. She was recognised as a warrior queen who protected men in battle and encouraged them to execute deeds of bravery.

More recently, the sexual overtones of the belly dance have contributed to the belief that it was its movements that gave the dance its poor reputation. This is a stigma that has persisted and has led those who take the dance seriously to reject the term 'belly dance', preferring to use such names as 'Danse du Ventre', 'Danse Oriental' and 'Raks Sharki' in the vain hope it would gain respectability.

For thousands of years the sexual connotations of belly dance have been prevalent. The dance has played an important role in fertility rituals, being performed as a means of sexual selection, and it has been closely associated with street dancers who have combined their dancing with prostitution.

For many centuries, the erotic aspects of the dance changed very little throughout the Arab world, despite the many attempts to clean up its image. Eventually, it evolved into a more sophisticated art form, the movements becoming more stylised, technical and less lascivious or erotic.

Despite the dance being constantly exploited and undermined it has successfully continued to survive and develop to become a popular form of entertainment in the West. In the Middle East and North Africa the dance has also retained its original significance in trance, ritual and fertility dances that are still performed by some people today.

In Egypt and surrounding areas, women continue to perform the belly dance at private parties on family occasions or at other festivities, although others sometimes frown on them for doing this. Nevertheless, for those brave enough to dance, the spontaneous and improvised movements give them an opportunity to express their frustration, vitality, sexuality and sensuality with joyous abandon.

The Zar

Today, women in the Sudan and in the Middle East, when feeling unhappy or unwell, take part in the psychotherapeutic cult of the Zar. As well as providing entertainment, here dance is used as part of a religious ceremony. Under the guidance of the group leader or sheikha az-aar, and using incense and massage and drumming from dawn until dusk, often for days, the participants find spiritual fulfilment and a means of obliging or exorcising the demons which they believe to have possessed them, causing their illness. In Morocco, the Zar cult is called the 'Hadra', meaning right of exorcism, and it is older than Islam, working around and through Islamic law rather than existing in competition with it. (Although the National Islamic Front's social programme aims to operate a clampdown on Zar practices, which often allow women greater freedom to smoke, drink and act out fantasies than they would otherwise exercise.)

Sometimes specialist dancers robed in white who have been possessed and healed are called upon to perform the Zar. Energetic male dancers, who leap, twist and turn, join them as they hold their arms up above their heads. As the specialist dancer performs movements of the traditional religious dance of the Muslim Brotherhood and becomes possessed, she is circled by a group of both male and female dancers. Her movements become less and less restrained, and the quickening pace and hypnotic beat of the music stimulate her until she finally collapses.

By freely improvising to the rhythmic drumming and chanting of male musicians, the women who take part in these rituals dance themselves into a trance-like state through which they identify and communicate with the demon that has possessed them. When they come out of their trance, they believe the demon spirit has left their body and that their sickness is healed. Sometimes animals are also sacrificed or gifts offered in an effort to placate the demons.

In spite of Egyptian Islamic fundamentalists' objections to this ritual dance, the cult of the Zar and its various ceremonies are still practised today. Women gather outside the Temple of Karnak to take part in the ceremony and also in towns and more remote areas in the countryside. These events are usually practised in the poorer neighbourhoods to prevent and discourage tourists from witnessing such occasions, as they are frowned upon by the Egyptian government that believes that western tourists will think less of the country if they see such practices.

In Saudi Arabia and many other areas of the Middle East, Zar cult ceremonies are also discouraged. They therefore have to be held discreetly, so the women have to gather in private whenever and wherever they can.

Belly Dance Styles

In the West, most of the belly dance styles performed today are based on the Ghawazee gypsy style that has been refined and modified. Although attempts have been made to carry on the traditional folk form, there is much less intensity and earthiness in the dance than previously.

One particular style, in which the movements are centred on the lower half of the body with the arms raised in a position similar to that of the Ghawazee, is known as the Baladi, or Baledi, which means in Egyptian 'of the country' or 'my people – my village'. The Baladi should be performed as a happy, lively joyous dance by a solo dancer entertaining guests attending weddings or other big celebrations.

Samia Gamal, a well-known Egyptian dancer of the 1930s and 1940s, incorporated ballet movements into the belly dance, creating her own unique style. A variation of her dance called Raks Sharki (meaning oriental dance) has recently emerged as an art form.

When I saw a performance of Raks Sharki many years ago, the movements of the dance appeared to be based on the isolation of the hips and upper torso and was danced mainly on the balls of the feet. It was very graceful, balletic and controlled, but lacked earthiness and a certain amount of sensuality.

Egyptian Raks Sharki dance movements, which I was introduced to by a male teacher in Egypt, had balletic elements and were often based on the flat of the foot, including wide steps, hip drops and pushes. It is a style that has recently become very popular in the West.

Many students in the UK believe that the style of Raks Sharki that has been prevalent over the last thirty years is the only authentic form of Egyptian dance and that all other forms taught are wrong. This is not so. In fact, the dance does not portray a true interpretation of the style of Egyptian dance that has been in existence for thousands of years and which is preferred by Egyptians. Sadly, the attitude of some Raks Sharki teachers and students has caused a great division in the world of oriental dance between those who support the idea that Raks Sharki is the 'true' belly dance and those that think otherwise. It has created a 'them' and 'us' situation which myself and many others find totally unacceptable and unnecessary. In my opinion there is no right or wrong way to perform the belly dance, whatever an individual's choice, it should be accepted and respected with tolerance – and it might be useful to keep this in mind when you are trying out the dance movements introduced in Chapter 7. However, before moving on to the practical guide to belly dance, a brief look at the health benefits of belly dance is included by way of introduction to the physical side of the dance and its benefits.

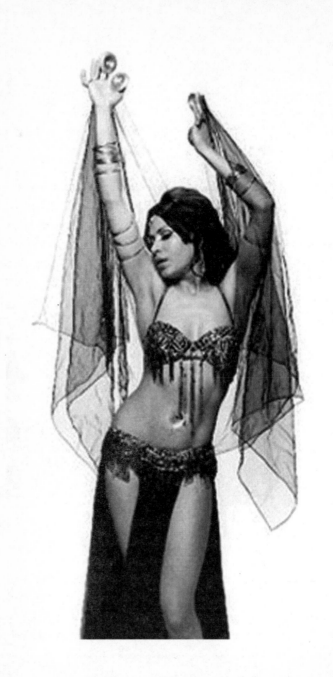

6

Belly Dancing for Health and Life

Through the sacred power of the belly dance, the dance of mother earth, we re-awaken our inner selves and regain the spiritual energies of the body, mind and soul. Belly dancing enables women to re-establish the lost link to their creativity, from which many have been disconnected for centuries. Unlike ballet and other forms of exercise and dance that impose movements upon the individual, the movements of this ancient dance are created by the intrinsic power within each individual.

Many women who attend belly dancing classes do so for health benefits and relaxation. They may want to get fit after surgery, ease lower back pain, ease suffering from the early stages of arthritis or multiple sclerosis, improve their co-ordination and balance or simply boost their energy levels.

Benefits of Belly Dancing Classes

Belly dancing can be enjoyed by anyone aged from three to ninety-three. A dancer does not require a size eight figure or a perfect torso to look good and accomplished. Unfortunately, women in the West have been conditioned by the media to believe that their bodies should look thin and svelte, and because they find it impossible to achieve this image, they become dissatisfied with themselves and feel inferior, unfulfilled and frustrated.

You do not have to be slim to become a belly dancer. Actually, the more voluptuous and fleshy the women, the more sensually they seem to move. In my experience, larger women make beautiful dancers. I have always encouraged my larger students to make the most of what they have.

Belly dancing can help to change how a woman thinks about herself. By gradually encouraging students to become aware of their negative attitudes to themselves and at the same time to think positively about what they have achieved and can achieve in the future, they begin to accept that it is possible to feel comfortable with their own bodies. This in turn helps the women to regain their self-confidence and reach the full potential of their vitality and sensuality through dance.

During exercise, stress is reduced as a result of the increase in blood flow to the brain and to the muscles. This in turn stimulates the production of naturally occurring chemical compounds called endorphins and encephalins. They have pain-relieving properties and effects resembling those of morphine or other opiates. They also create a rise in energy levels which in turn improves physical activity, lessens tension and depression and relaxes muscle tension. There is no doubt that freeing the body from restricted movement eliminates anxiety, improves mobility and frees the spirit. This creates a substantial feeling of physical and spiritual well being and enhances the quality of life.

Ill Health

The belly dance is a wonderful form of exercise for women suffering from digestive problems and irritable bowel syndrome (IBS). One woman I know of who suffered from these ailments and whose problem had been diagnosed as a stress condition found that her digestive problems, IBS and stress totally disappeared after attending a course of lessons.

A different student of mine who attended classes, told me her life was made wretched as a result of the early stages of endometriosis, a problem suffered by women where the presence of tissue similar to the lining of the uterus is found at sites other than the uterus. She benefited greatly by concentrating on movements of the pelvic region. Consequently, her health and life style dramatically improved. She was even more delighted when she discovered she was expecting a baby, after having unsuccessfully tried to conceive for several years.

Lack of freedom of movement places an enormous amount of stress and strain on body, mind and spirit. Ill health is often the result of the body's reaction to stress, which can block energy flow and may result in stomach problems. If stomach problems persist they can lead to continuous indigestion, IBS, diarrhoea and possible vomiting.

Movement improves muscle tone and tightens up important muscles, particularly those that surround and support the internal organs and those which help to stretch and strengthen the pelvic floor. During exercise muscles contract so the more we demand from our muscles, the stronger they become. Stress can cause a shortening of some muscles that could affect the entire structure of our bodies so it is very important to keep the muscle tone and strength to maintain correct posture and good health.

Tense muscles can affect posture and may also be related to other discomforts such as backache, neckache, gynaecological problems, headaches, insomnia, depression, irritability and premature ageing. Such problems can greatly affect our outlook on life, as well as our quality of life, affecting our relationships, emotions, attitudes and everyday situations.

The function of the muscles is to move the joints, which are attached to the end of the bones by ligaments. The bone ends are protected by articular cartilage and a capsule with a synovial membrane encloses the whole. The synovial membrane secretes the lubricating synovial fluid, a thick, colourless lubricating and nourishing fluid surrounding the joints that allows them to move smoothly.

Synovial membranes are self-lubricating as they provide their own fluid but the synovial fluid can only be produced if there is movement between two bones. If there is no movement, the fluid will not be produced and the joints will become dry and stiff. So if you start moving your joints gently you will produce synovial fluid.

Arthritis is a very common complaint, affecting people of all ages. Arthritic students greatly benefit from attending belly dancing classes because movement helps keep the joints fully mobile, enabling them to increase self-lubrication. Lack of gentle exercise prevents the joints from carrying out their full range of movement. Movement is extremely important in preventing deterioration of the joints which, if neglected, in time will lead to more serious problems.

Back pain is a condition that affects a great number of people often simply through ignorance. It is very important to become aware of your physical and mental condition and to help yourself by paying attention to your diet, the exercise you take, your daily routine and other aspects of life such as relationships and work.

Back pain is very common, a major reason for this being that often the back is not being used properly. This is frequently a result of poor posture or because chairs, car seats and mattresses do not give the back the adequate support required. Another cause of back pain is lifting and carrying objects incorrectly and exercising too vigorously.

If the spine is slightly out of alignment this may also cause back pain. In this instance it is definitely worth visiting a chiropractor or osteopath who can realign your spine and help relieve the back pain, as well as other discomforts. Even an aching knee can be attributed to a back problem.

Pain is also caused because people do not use their backs sufficiently. Lack of movement can cause the back to stiffen and then become painful. When performing the gentle rocking and circular movement of the belly dance, this stimulates the back muscles, which increases the suppleness in the back muscles. This alleviates stiffness which in turn helps to relieve lower back pain.

Some students have suffered from what is commonly termed a slipped disc. This is a misnomer – there is actually no such thing. Movement cannot dislodge the discs themselves as they are strongly attached to the two vertebrae they sit between. What happens is that the disc leaks its pulpy nucleus into the vertebral cavity, and presses on a nerve. This problem can be caused by a sudden awkward movement and can be very painful. The best course of treatment is gentle manipulation with a physiotherapist, osteopath or chiro-practor. This treatment will help to unlock the joint that has become jammed. Once it has been treated and provided there are no serious problems, you should be able to follow up the treatment with some gentle belly dance movements. If you do suffer from severe back pain, however, always consult your doctor before attending classes in belly dancing.

Many back sufferers believe that the correct thing to do to ease their back pain is to get plenty of bed rest. Whilst in some cases this is advisable, it is not always the right thing to do, as not moving the back can sometimes cause stiffening.

Frozen shoulder is a common disorder of the shoulder joint, which becomes increasingly painful and stiff, restricting movement of the shoulder. The condition may develop following injury or for no apparent reason. It can be extremely distressing and in some cases debilitating. Treatment involving gentle stretching movements will help restore some space to the joint, so that the head of the humerus (the bone of the upper arm) has room to manoeuvre.

If you suffer from a frozen shoulder, only exercise with caution. Do seek advice from a practitioner, who will be able to recommend a programme of corrective treatment and exercise. While it is painful it is not advisable to do any elevation or shoulder shimmies but you will be able to do many other dance movements in class.

Sciatica is a pain felt in the back, outer side of the thigh, leg and bottom and sometimes in the sole of the foot. It is usually associated with a back problem. The pain may start suddenly, brought on by lifting something awkwardly or by a twisting movement. There may be numbness and weakness in one leg. If the pain persistently occurs it is advisable to see your doctor as soon as possible, who should refer you to a physiotherapist. Alternatively, contact your local chiropractor or osteopath directly and they will administer appropriate treatment.

Correct posture is most important to maintain a feeling of well being but it is something that is seldom attained throughout our lives. Poor posture that goes unchecked limits the mobility of the spine and strains the skeleton, often leading to further pain and discomfort.

For some people, bad posture can be caused by psychological problems, injury or the fact that the back is out of alignment. Stretching and strengthening exercises will help to counteract poor posture. If you suffer from persistent pain, before starting any dance or fitness programme, seek advice from a therapist, otherwise you may further aggravate your problem.

Incorrect posture such as rounded shoulders, head jutting forward and a dropped rib cage can cause muscle strain and backache, produce a bulging belly and other discomforts because of the imbalance of the body. Poor posture can be improved but it is no easy task to change the bad habits of a lifetime.

There are five common types of bad posture. The first occurs when the back is too straight and has insufficient curve. The second, the 'hollow back,' which involves inward curvature of the spine, is known as lordosis. The third, scoliosis, is a sideways deviation of the spine. The fourth, a jutting out of the spine known as 'poke neck', causes a nasty ache across the shoulders and base of the neck. Finally, bad posture can be caused by a rounded thorax and shoulders.

Breathing Correctly

Correct breathing is fundamental to our sense of well being. If we do not breathe properly, the body will not get the full amount of oxygen it requires in order to function as it should. Incorrect breathing leads to many problems such as tension, poor circulation, headaches, digestive problems, lack of concentration and energy. Most of us tend to breathe all the time from the chest, taking short, shallow breaths as though we are constantly exerting ourselves physically or in a permanent state of anger, fear or anxiety. We do not breathe deeply from the abdomen, the part of the body cavity below the chest. Abdominal breathing that promotes relaxation should occur for most of the time when we are relaxed. Unfortunately, those who live with permanent anxiety, tension and stress seem to have forgotten how to breathe abdominally and this may have to be consciously relearned.

The essence of correct breathing is to exercise the diaphragm, which is the muscular partition between the chest and the abdomen. When you breathe in, the diaphragm, which is a dome-like shape, causes the rib cage to descend and expand, increasing the chest capacity and enabling you to take in the maximum amount of air. This in turn pushes the abdominal organs down causing them to swell.

As you pull your stomach in, the diaphragm is raised. This helps you to expel the stale air in your lungs, thus increasing your oxygen supply, stimulating your blood circulation and strengthening weak and flabby stomach muscles.

You may find the method of correct breathing difficult at first, as it is not what many of us think of as deep breathing. If, however, you make a determined effort and persevere with this method of breathing, it will soon become automatic and you will not need to think about it any more. Breathing deeply will help to reduce tension and stress and will provide you with more energy and a feeling of well being.

Try the following breathing technique slowly, and, most importantly, only when you have warmed up, as breathing exercises of this kind can be quite strenuous.

As you breathe in, push your stomach out, and as you breathe out, pull your stomach in. To begin with, only do four or five of these breathing exercises at a time, as you may feel a little light-headed. Once you have become accustomed to breathing in this way, you should be able to do it continually. It is a great exercise to help to tone up abdominal muscles and prevent a flabby stomach from developing.

Movements of the dance

Through the movements of the belly dance blocked energy is released. This frees the body from both mental and physical tension, enabling it to function more effectively.

The movements of belly dancing (some of which are introduced in Chapter 7) are based on the structure of the body, so there is no stress or strain for those of you wishing to start a programme of exercise after injury or illness. You should, however, only take lessons if your medical support team agrees to your doing so.

Muscles work in groups. When they are not used they become weak and lose their elasticity and strength, in which case they have to be retrained to function effectively. If you discipline your muscles steadily and to their full capacity, through gentle exercise, your flexibility will improve considerably.

It is important to understand the difference between a tense group of muscles and a relaxed group of muscles and to be able to feel each group of muscles move independently from other groups. Isolating the groups of muscles correctly should enable you to move one group of muscles without moving another.

If isolation is performed correctly you should be able to move the upper part of the torso without moving the lower half and vice versa. To isolate correctly, raise your rib cage, gently drop your shoulders and relax your knees. From a standing position you should now be able to slide your rib cage from side to side without moving your hips or move your hips without moving your upper torso.

Dance movements that concentrate on the lower region of the body release the energy block of the solar plexus situated between the twelfth thoracic vertebrae and the first lumber vertebrae. Shamans discovered that by reactivating this area of the body, the effect on illness was very positive, especially on diseases of the stomach.

It is most important that your basic stance is correct, particularly before starting with an exercise or dance movement. Many teachers know little about correct posture and are therefore not able to correct their students' faults. Therefore, students tend to dance with their knees bent too much, with rounded shoulders, dropped rib cage or hunched shoulders – all of which are likely to cause problems.

When the knees are bent too much the line of gravity does not fall correctly. The knees should only bend to five degrees of friction, that is, just be slightly flexed. The feet should be held to the floor, the rib cage elevated and the shoulders down and relaxed. If you stand in this manner, your spine will be correctly aligned.

There are three points of support in the feet, which are on the first and fifth metatarsi (the bones of the foot that connect the ankle to the toes) and on the heel. If these three points are held to the floor, the knees flexed to five degrees and the rib cage elevated, the line of gravity goes upward towards the shoulders. The spine is then held in its correct position and relaxed.

Standing or dancing with knees locked may cause lordosis in the back, a contraction of the lumber vertebrae that forces the back inward. If you keep your knees locked you will not have an open back or freedom of movement in the pelvic region and will therefore find many of the dance movements difficult to do.

Throwing the knee outwards when attempting particular movements is also a bad habit that is seldom corrected by teachers. This is usually done when the hips are rotated in a backward motion, for example when performing a figure of eight or bouncing the hips backwards. Throwing the knee out can damage muscles in the groin, causing abductus muscle strain. This is a common injury, particularly with sports people and dancers, which can be debilitating and take a long time to heal. To prevent this occurring you should only push the hip back gently, as fast as it will go without any strain, making sure the knee is flexible and held directly over the foot. If you hold the leg correctly in this position, as well as preventing groin strain, you will find your hips will have much more freedom of movement and will enable you to do the movements without any difficulty

I get many students who complain that they have never been able to do certain movements without difficulty. By making sure they have the correct posture and that they are holding their legs in the correct position they find that they can do the movements effortlessly, much to their surprise.

Unfortunately, many teachers lack teaching skills and are not proficient in every aspect of Middle Eastern dance. More worryingly, they may have little or no knowledge of medical problems that may occur or the various types of poor posture they are likely to come across when teaching. Therefore, they are not able to advise or correct their students. If you attend a class where posture and other bad habits go uncorrected you should leave it, for you could risk injury that may eventually lead to long term problems.

Sitting or standing with the legs crossed or close together may also damage muscles. Ideally, the thighs should be kept open but because of our upbringing most of us keep our legs closed or crossed. In this way as soon as we push our thighs together we damage muscles that move one part of the body away from another, known as abductors, which then become over-stretched. To avoid this happening, whenever possible, sit with your knees open.

Some students, when belly dancing for the first time, experience low back pain. The reason for this is that the sacrum, which is part of the backbone, has not been used to its full potential. Through the movements of the dance, you will start to use the sacral vertebrae correctly, and this may cause a little strain and lower back pain. If the pain persists when dancing, it is advisable to seek medical advice.

When dancing, many students become anxious when they experience a clicking noise in their hips or knees. This is caused by bubbles in the synovial fluid popping and is like a release of air from a vacuum but is nothing to worry about. The remedy is a good massage.

Occasionally I have students who complain of a crunching sensation in their hips when doing the dance movements. This could be a sign of the early stages of arthritis. If you experience this, seek medical advice.

Conclusion

Why should you or anyone else wish to take up belly dancing? Why does it attract people from all walks of life? Apart from its fascinating history and the immense benefits in terms of health and fitness, if you are a person who loves dance and are seeking something truly different that embodies all the qualities and emotion that we imagine dance should evoke, then this is what you are looking for: the dance of mother earth.

Whether learning the movements of the dance for health reasons, for relaxation or perhaps because you want to become a professional dancer under expert guidance, learning the dance of mother earth is a highly enjoyable way to harmonise your body, mind, soul and spirit to heal and balance yourself. Dance is a spiritual channel and through this sacred dance we re-awaken our inner selves and regain our spirituality and life-giving power, for all things are born of women through the life-giving power of mother earth.

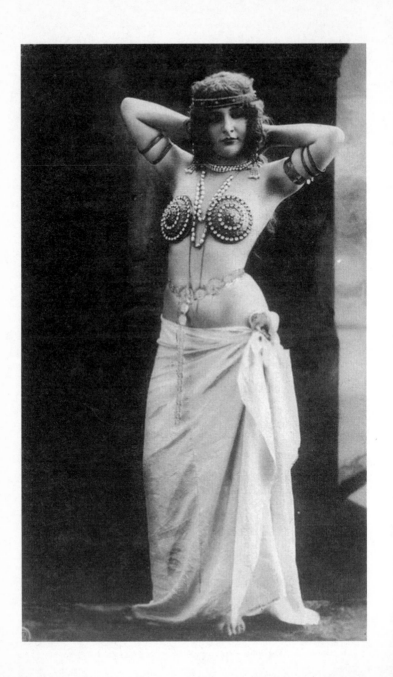

7

Dance Movements

Basic

As a practical introduction to belly dance this chapter provides a step-by-step guide to ten basic movements before progressing to include in greater detail a guide to some of the more advanced movements. There are also suggestions for ways to combine movements as with increased confidence you may wish to create your own moves and routines.

Before attempting any of the movements, however, it is essential that the correct standing position is assumed as follows:

(i) Elevate rib cage.
(ii) Bend knees slightly.
(iii) Keep feet firmly on the floor.
(iv) Relax shoulders and hold the head up.

When you feel entirely comfortable with your starting position you are ready to begin the first movement.

Movement 1 – Basic Hip Rotation

(i) Hold your arms out to the side with elbows about waist

level and with palms facing either up or down.

(ii)   Stick your bottom out and roll your hips over to the right.

(iii) Then push your hips forward as far as you can and roll them over to the left.

(iv)   Push your hips back and immediately roll them over to the right.

(v)   Once more push your hips forward as far as you can and continue to rotate them in a circle several times.

This movement may be repeated by rotating the hips in the opposite direction or varied by the accompaniment of arm movements as follows:

(i)   Place your arms by your sides.

(ii)   Bring them forward so that your elbows are level with your waist.

(iii) Place your hands back-to-back so that your wrists face outwards and so your hands are held just below the level of your navel.

(iv)   Whilst completing the hip rotation gently move your arms around your body until they are behind you, keeping level with your bottom.

(v)   Repeat this movement in a continual motion, slowly bringing the arms forward again and then back as you rotate your hips.

A further variant on the hip rotation is to rotate the hips in the same direction twice before changing to the opposite direction. Alternatively, you may like to try rotating the hips in a very large circle followed by a rotation of two smaller circles, or experiment with other similar combinations of variants in circle size such as rotating your hips in a small circular motion several times to the right and then several times to the left.

Movement 2 – Pelvic Roll

(i)   Assume starting position.

(ii)   Stand with feet spread apart to align with the hips.

(iii) Stick your bottom out as far as possible and slowly roll the hips over to the right.

(iv)   Now stick your bottom out again and slowly roll your hips over to the left.

(v)   Repeat several times pushing the hips from right to left and back in a continuous rolling motion (like you are performing half a hip rotation, omitting the movement in front of the body).

This movement can be performed in reverse by doing it in front of the body, remembering to push hips forward as far as possible. The pelvic roll can also be turned into a more advanced dance movement by using the feet at the same time. This is achieved as follows:

(i)   Stand with feet apart at hip width.

(ii)   Whilst rolling the hips over to the right raise your left heel.

(iii) Once the hips are over to the right lower the left heel.

(iv)   This time roll your hips over to the left at which point raise your right heel.

(v)   Lower the right heel before rolling your hips back over to the right.

(vi)   Repeat several times.

You might also like to try accompanying this dance movement with a basic position for the arms, raising them out to the side with elbows relaxed and held at waist level. It should be noted that when arms are held out to the front or at your side they should never be raised above shoulder height.

Movement 3 – Basic Right and Left Hip Rolls

Whilst doing this next movement it is extremely important that the knee is not swung out to the side or turned inwards but held as steady as possible over the foot. This is not only to ensure that the movement is performed correctly but also to prevent groin strain.

(i)   Assume start position.

(ii)   Place your right leg slightly forward.

(iii)   Raise the right heel, bend the right knee and keep the left knee flexed.

(iv)   Whilst keeping the right heel up and the knee bent rotate the right hip in a circle several times.

(v)   Repeat the movement by rotating the hip in the opposite direction several times, then relax.

(vi)   Now place your left leg forward.

(vii)   Raise your left heel, bend your left knee and keep your right knee flexed.

(viii) Whilst keeping the left heel up and the knee bent rotate your left hip in a circle several times.

(ix)   Repeat the movement by rotating the hip in the opposite direction several times, then relax.

As with previous movements, a variation can be produced by using one large circle followed by two smaller circles for both the right and left hip rolls featured here. An undulating version can also be performed as follows:

(i)   Assume starting position.

(ii)   Slowly rotate the right hip in a large circle.

(iii)   Then, whilst performing the smaller rotations, bend both knees, remembering to keep your back straight at all times.

(iv) Straighten up from this position smoothly and slowly and immediately repeat the movement by slowly rotating the right hip, then bend both knees throughout the smaller and quicker rotations of the right hip.

(v) Repeat several times then perform the movement on the left side.

As an accompanying arm movement raise your right arm when the right leg is forward, bending it gently from the elbow so that the arm is curved above the head, but holding your left arm by your side, rounded at the elbow so that the hand is pointing towards the left hip and the arm is framing the left hip. (Once again reverse this procedure when performing the rotation movement on the opposite side.)

Movement 4 – Circle Within a Circle and Combinations
During this highly popular movement the feet should be spread apart, placed flat on the floor and remain parallel throughout.

The basic step

(i) Stand with the feet spread apart to align with the hips and flex the knees.

(ii) Take a very small step forward onto the flat of the right foot and at the same time pivot slightly on your left foot to the left.

(iii) Continue stepping on to the flat of the right foot until you have made a full circle on the spot and are facing forward once more.

The basic step in conjunction with the hip circle (i.e. 'circle within a circle')

(i)   Repeat as above but in this instance as you step onto the flat of the right foot stick your bottom out.

(ii)   Roll your hips over to the right, push them forward and then roll them over to the left, making a full circular movement of the hip as with the basic hip rotation.

(iii) On completion of this first circle, stick your bottom out again as you take another small step forward onto the flat of the right foot and follow this with a further circle of the hips.

(iv) Continue the movement as in (ii) then repeat this several times until you have completed a circle on the spot.

Once you have got the hang of this movement it should be tried on the left side and also in conjunction with arm movements as used with the basic hip rotation.

Movement 5 – Pelvic Tilts.
This pelvic tilt is one of the best movements for easing lower back pain and strengthening the pelvic floor as it basically involves the repeated motion of pushing your bottom out to tilt your pelvis back before thrusting it forward and upward in a gentle rocking movement. As this move is fairly self-explanatory, I will focus on some variations for you to try once you have practised the pelvic tilt in its basic form.

Undulating Pelvic Tilt

(i) Tilt your pelvis forward and back four times whilst bending both knees, then forward and back again four times whilst straightening up until your knees are only slightly bent, taking care to keep the knees flexible rather than locking them. Repeat several times.

Travelling Pelvic Tilt

(i) Assume starting position.
(ii) As you take a very short step forward onto the flat of the right foot tilt your pelvis back and forward, then repeat this with a step forward onto the left foot.
(iii) Continue tilting pelvis back and forth whilst alternating small steps forward on the right and left foot.

Arm movements to accompany the Pelvic Tilt

(i) Place arms at your sides.
(ii) Raise arms up in front of torso no higher than the bust, relaxing the elbows and raising the hands.
(iii) Whilst performing the pelvic tilts roll the hands outwards until the palms face up then roll them inwards until the palms face the floor.

Movement 6 – The Basic Hip Drop.

(i) Stand with feet close together but not touching and knees flexed.
(ii) Raise the right heel and bend the right knee, ensuring that the left knee remains flexed throughout the movement and does not lock.
(iii) Push the right hip down towards the floor then raise and repeat several times, saying to yourself, 'Down, up, down, up…' as an aide towards achieving a suitable rhythm.

A useful tip to remember is that this movement can be made easier by placing your hands on your hips so that each time you drop your right hip you can push it down with the right hand, and likewise with the left.

In terms of possible variations on this move you can twist

each hip forward before dropping and then raising it. Otherwise try a double hip drop, dropping and raising the right hip twice in succession before pushing it back, then repeating this again before changing to the left hip. In this instance, you may find it useful repeating the words, 'Forward, drop, drop, back, drop, drop…' to keep a steady rhythm going and if you wish to include arms movements use those recommended for the pelvic tilt.

To perform alternate hip drops push one hip down at a time and then the other to produce a smooth and fairly swift movement. This variation is well-suited to a slightly more adventurous arm movement, achieved by raising both arms above the head and then dropping them at the elbows, keeping the hands up. You should either hold this position throughout or, for greater variety, turn both hands in and then out at the same time rotating the hands from the wrist.

Movement 7 – Forward Step Back Step
To next try something a little different and increase the range of types of basic moves so far covered, this movement concentrates primarily on footwork. To avoid straining ankle-joints remember that a warm-up is always advisable.

(i)   Assume starting position.
(ii)   Flex the knees and keep feet close together but not touching.
(iii)   Step forward onto the flat of the right foot.
(iv)   Keeping the left foot where it is, raise it slightly off the floor then immediately lower it to the floor.
(v)   Step back onto the flat of the right foot and raise and lower the left foot again.
(vi)   Continue by stepping forward onto the flat of the right foot.

Once this basic step has been mastered try pushing out your right hip as you step forward and back on your right foot, and likewise, when you try the move on your left side, push the left hip out as you move the left foot forward and back. It should be noted that this step can also be performed on the balls of the feet, though care must be taken to ensure the heels do not drop.

Movement 8 – Hip Twist Walk

(i)   Assume starting position but stand with your feet close together.

(ii) Raise up onto the balls of both feet, take small alternate steps forward and practice walking around the room on the balls of your feet.

(iii) To add the hip twist, as you step forward onto the ball of the right foot twist your right hip forward, then repeat this with the left before continuing to step and twist your hips alternately as you travel forward.

This movement should be performed with arms held out to the side, keeping them below shoulder level with elbows relaxed, hands raised and palms facing the floor as you travel forward.

Movement 9 – Travelling Hip Push

As this movement involves a side-to-side push of the hips whilst you travel forward it is tempting to actually step forward but in order to complete the move correctly you must step from side-to-side (from right to left).

(i)   Assume starting position.

(ii) Stand with your feet close together and with knees flexed.

(iii) As you step to the right onto the flat of the right foot immediately raise the left foot slightly off the floor and bring it towards the right foot.

(iv) Similarly, as you step to the left onto the flat of the left foot immediately raise your right foot slightly off the floor and bring it towards your left foot.

(v) Now try to push your hips from side-to-side as you do this walk, pushing your right hip out to the side as you step to the right and left hip out to the side as you step to the left.

(vi) Continue to practice this move on the flat of your feet until you feel sufficiently confident to try it on the balls of your feet.

Eventually you'll find yourself able to push the hips from left to right with little effort and at this point it might be fun to try travelling backwards on the flat of the feet then up on the balls of the feet. Hold the arms in the standard position out in front throughout, no higher than bust level and with hands raised.

Movement 10 – Travelling Hip Drops.

This lively dance movement requires the use of three different dance steps simultaneously and so may be found to be the most complex of these ten introductory movements. However, it is still fairly basic and should not present too many problems.

(i) Stand with feet close together but not touching.

(ii) Whilst stepping back onto the flat of the right foot simultaneously raise the left heel and drop the left hip twice in quick succession.

(iii) Quickly step back onto the flat of the left foot, immediately raise your right heel and drop the right hip twice in quick succession. (When performing this movement do not move the foot that is placed in front with the heel raised or this will create an extra step and be out of rhythm – just raise the heel and bounce your hips.)

To conclude this section here are a few final suggestions for ways to vary the travelling hip drops. Firstly, follow the instructions for the basic movement but instead of doing two hip drops on the right and two on the left, twist your right hip forward and bounce it twice before pulling it back and bouncing it twice – and then repeat for the left hip. At this point you should have completed four hip bounces for each side but you could double the amount if preferred and do four bounces in front and four pulled back for each hip. Accompany the move with the arms by raising them up above your head, relaxed at the elbows, swaying them over to the right when you start to drop your hips on the right side and over to the left when you drop your hips left.

Advanced

In this section you will be introduced to some of the slightly more advanced movements and so it is advisable to make sure you are proficient in performing the ten basic moves before progressing to this section. The first movement we will tackle is, however, intended to be gentle rather than vigorous, which should ease the transition to more complex movements.

Movement 11 – Figure Eight and Variations.
The figure eight is a smooth, graceful and sensual movement of the hips which can be performed to a slow or medium tempo.

(i)   Assume starting position but standing with your feet slightly apart.
(ii) Flex the knees, keeping them as still as possible, and hold the feet firmly to the floor.
(iii) Push the right hip forward and out then push back the right hip and back again.

(iv) Hold the right hip where it is whilst you push the left hip forward and out and then push back again as with the right hip.

(v) Hold the left hip back as you push the right hip out then back.

(vi) Repeat several times.

For variations on this move you can try the reverse figure eight which requires that the hips are moved in the opposite direction to the standard figure eight. It is important at all times that the knees are kept flexed and not bent or moved to and fro. Alternatively, to perform a vertical figure eight raise your heels as you raise your hips, in order to lift them up higher, and bringing the hip and heel down at the same time. The undulating figure eight can be achieved by doing four figure eights whilst slowly bending your knees and then another four as you straighten up again. To avoid back strain and achieve good posture it is important to keep the back straight whilst executing this move so avoid leaning forward whilst bending the knees and keep your arms out to the sides, below shoulder level and with elbows relaxed, to aid balance.

The oriental arm movement is a graceful accompaniment you might like to include once you feel able, as follows:

(i) Place your arms down by your sides.

(ii) Push your elbows out so that your arms are rounded.

(iii) Raise your right shoulder, followed by your right elbow and finally bring your hand up and bend the arm fully at the elbow.

(iv) As you bend the right arm at the elbow do the same movement on the left side and then continue the movement by raising the arms alternately.

Movement 12 – Camel Rock.

This is again a rather gentle movement, which involves a graceful rocking motion of the hips achieved by shifting weight from one leg to another as you step forward. If you've ever ridden a camel you should be familiar with the rocking motion that characterizes the animal's walk but it is otherwise no tricky feat to imagine the slow and lazy pace determined by a continual shift of weight from one side to the other.

(i)   Assume standing position, this time standing with the feet close together but not touching.

(ii) Elevate the rib cage and hold this position throughout the movement. Place your hands behind you and rest them gently on your bottom with palms facing outwards.

(iii) As you step forward onto the flat of the right foot simultaneously contract your abdomen and stick your bottom out.

(iv) Immediately relax your abdomen and tilt your pelvis up forward and up.

(vi) Continue by stepping forward again onto the flat of the right foot, then again on the flat of the left foot, and so forth.

For a first shot at varying the camel rock, try taking double steps, first to the right and then to the left, as you rock your hips. Rather than simply stepping out and back with the right foot, as with previous moves, this should involve your stepping back on to the left foot following each step out on to the right. To get the rocking motion right, each time you step out with either right or left foot, you should simultaneously contract your abdomen and stick your bottom out, then immediately relax your abdomen and tilt your pelvis forward and up – twice for each step. It may help to say, 'step and step,' to the count of one and two. Continue alternating on each foot whilst stepping slightly to the right and then to the left as you go.

A further variation on the camel rock is to perform the move turning on the spot instead of travelling forward, either using the flats of the feet or stepping up onto the balls of the feet. Suggested arm movements include placing your arms behind your back and resting the back of the hands gently on your bottom. For a more dramatic performance you could try placing your right hand at your temple as you travel to the right, with your left arms out to the left with elbow relaxed, and reverse this as you travel to the left, with left hand on left temple.

Movement 13 – The Hip Shimmy.

This is one of the most important of all the belly dance moves, used widely and often in combination with other dance steps. It may take some time to perfect but is more than worth persevering with as the perfect shimmy is an essential component of any worthy belly dance.

(i) Assume the start position, with feet set close together firmly on the ground and knees flexed. (Whilst first practising the shimmy place your hands firmly together as though in prayer as this will stop other parts of the body from moving – particularly your hands, arms and shoulders.)

(ii) Drop your bottom slightly, as though you are about to sit down but have changed your mind.

(iii) Very slightly twist your right hip forward.

(iv) Push the right hip back and simultaneously move the left hip forward.

(v) Push the left hip back and simultaneously move the right hip forward.

This movement should be done extremely quickly in order to achieve the hip shimmy, by alternating the hips forward and back in rapid succession to music of a very fast tempo. As a variant, whilst doing the basic hip shimmy twist the right hip forward to a count of four and then the left, also to a count of four, or try this with a count of two – ensuring that you keep shimmying!

Another fun way to shimmy is to do it whilst 'travelling'. First try lifting the feet whilst shimmying on the spot, then travel around the room taking small alternate steps, either on the flat or on the balls of your feet depending on how well practised you are. The shimmy can also be used with the basic hip twist introduced earlier to produce a hip twist walk with shimmy, either on the flats or the balls of the feet. A hip push shimmy combines this move with a more vigorous push of the hips out from side to side, executed as a travelling hip push shimmy (which should be self-explanatory) or a double hip push shimmy. For the double hip shimmy, take a small step on to the right foot, then bring the left foot up to it, before taking another step to the right. Then repeat this on the left side, stepping on to the flat of the left foot, bringing the right foot up to it and stepping out with the left again. To add the double hip pushes, each time you transfer your weight onto the flat of each foot push out the hip twice from the same side. The step pattern is as follows:

Right left. Right.   Left right. Left.
Push and push.   Push and push.

Once these side steps with hip pushes have been mastered, add the shimmy, try the movement on the flats and the balls of the feet, and experiment with travelling forward and backwards. At all times, however, keep your feet parallel moving them from side to side only and making sure you do not step directly forward at any point.

Movement 14 – Spins and Variations.

When practicing the spins extra care must be taken as you may experience dizziness, become disorientated and loose your balance. If at all possible it is advisable that these movements are practised with a friend or colleague for safety reasons although once you have mastered spins you should find that dizziness does not occur.

The basic spin is the best place to start.

(i)   First, try spinning to the right whilst keeping your right foot flat on the floor and raise your left heel.

(ii) Then, holding your right arms out in front and with the hand facing upwards, start to slowly spin to the right whilst looking hard and with concentration at your hand.

(iii) Slowly increase the speed of your spin, continuing to concentrate on your hand as this should reduce and hopefully eliminate dizziness. It is sensible to try this also in the opposite direction as it is likely that you will find spins easier on one side than on the other.

Variations on the spin include spinning whilst doing the hip shimmy, a highly effective movement that requires considerable practice but is well worth the effort. More flexible dancers might also like to try bending to the right as they shimmy to the right, repeating this on the left side also. The standard arm position for the spin is to raise the right arm when spinning to the right, so that it is held above the head, bent at the elbow to form a graceful curve. The left arm should instead be positioned at your side with the elbow pushing the arm out into a gentle curve also. Once you have performed a spin in this fashion change the arms and try the spin in the opposite direction.

Movement 15 – Upper Torso Circle and Combinations.

(i)   Assume starting position, standing with feet apart at hip width, flexing the knees.

(ii)   Bend to the right, then swing your upper torso forward, down, then over to the left and up.

(iii) Arch the back as far as possible, then swing over to the right and continue to do another one or two upper torso circles.

Follow this through by repeating the movement in the opposite direction and if feeling especially adventurous you could combine the move with a hip rotation by rotating the opposite hip to whichever side of the torso you are circling. Otherwise try a double upper torso circle by circling the torso twice in quick succession and perhaps try also using a combination of one large circle followed by two small circles in rapid succession. In addition, those who are highly flexible may like to experiment with brushing the floor with their hair in the traditionally flamboyant style of all good belly dancers!

Movement 16 – Circle within a Circle Combinations.

In this movement we will build upon the techniques acquired earlier in Movement 4, 'Basic Circle within a Circle', here used to combine one large hip rotation with the immediate succession of two smaller rotations. This is harder to master than it may sound and is a source of frustration for many students but with practice you will find it possible and the perseverance is definitely worth it.

(i)   Assume starting position

(ii)   Stand with feet wide apart, no wider than hip width, parallel, and with knees flexed.

(iii) Practise the basic step first which involves raising the right foot slightly off the floor and swinging the left leg forward whilst pivoting to the left on the flat of the left foot. Step onto the flat of the left foot on completing the half turn, so that you are now facing the opposite direction with feet still set apart and parallel. Take two smaller steps forward onto the flat of the right foot as you pivot on the left so that you are now facing the front again.

(iv) Next add the hip rotation. To complete your half circle as you step forward stick your bottom out and make one big circle anti-clockwise with the hips, followed by two smaller circles to bring you back round to the front.

Do several of these movements to the right then repeat in the opposite direction, swinging the left foot forward whilst making one large circle clockwise. Try also a hip rotation involving a single, large pivoting circle instead of three smaller circles, performed whilst you turn. You may also wish to experiment with the addition of pelvic twists and/or hip drops which provide a slightly different take on the basic step.

Movement 17 – Travelling Hip Twists with a Forward Step Back.

With this movement we return to focus primarily on foot work once again.

(i) Assume start position, standing with feet close together and knees flexed

(ii) Place the right foot forward then raise both heels.

(iii) Do four hip twists travelling to the right and then two forward step back steps on your left foot.

(iv) Then starting with your left foot do four hip twists travelling to the left and two forward step back steps on your right foot, which should leave you now ready to travel to the right again. Repeat several times.

Movement 18 – Hip Twists Followed by a Spin.

(i)   Assume starting position but standing with feet close together.

(ii) Place your right foot forward then raise yourself up onto the balls of both feet.

(iii) Travelling to your right in a very large circle do sixteen hip twists. (Once these are completed, you should be back to your starting position, facing the front.)

(iv) Now spin to the right to eight counts or, if you're feeling energetic, spin to sixteen counts. Alternatively, spin to the right for eight counts then to the left for eight counts.

Repeat the combination to the left, starting with the hip twists then finishing with a spin.

Movement 19 – Rib Cage Slide and Other Rib Cage Movements.

Before you begin this move it is essential that you have your rib cage elevated, otherwise you will find it difficult to perform the sequence correctly.

(i)   Assume start position but standing with your feet slightly apart and with the knees flexed.

(ii) Tighten the muscles in your backside and place your hands on your hips.

(iii) Taking extreme care not to move your hips or raise your shoulders slide your rib cage over to the right and then over to the left.

(iv) Repeat several times then relax.

One variant on this move is the Travelling Rib Cage Slide

(otherwise known as Rib Cage Walk) which may require extra concentration when trying for the first time. It basically involves taking a small step forward onto the flat of the right foot before performing the rib cage slide to both sides, and then repeating this with a step onto the flat of the left foot.

To achieve a Rib Cage Lift you must, from the start position, raise your rib cage making sure you do not pull your shoulders back, push forward from your diaphragm, lift your rib cage and then lower it again. The same movement is called a Rib Cage Push when pushing your rib cage forward rather than up, again without pulling the shoulders back. Both the rib cage lift and push can be done travelling forward if, with each step you take, you either raise and lower the rib cage or push it out and back – depending on which move you choose.

A Rib Cage Roll is a combination of the Rib Cage Lift and the Rib Cage Push such that you push your Rib Cage forward and then lift it, before pulling it back in and pushing it down and then immediately pushing it forward again to repeat the move several times. With a Travelling Rib Cage Roll, which is a very gentle, sensuous and snake-like movement that should become effortless with practice, you should find your hips simultaneously rolling back and forth as with the Camel Rock. As you step onto the flat of the right foot complete a rib cage roll simultaneously, then step onto the flat of the left foot and do another rib cage roll. Repeat several times.

You may also like to try a Rib Cage Circle or Rib Cage Figure Eight, which involves sliding and pushing the rib cage such that it traces each of these shapes respectively. Whilst this is to be encouraged, as both are difficult and challenging moves that should be fun to try and master, it is essential that you 'isolate' correctly which means that you must not move the lower part of your body as you move the top half or vice versa.

Movement 20 – Abdominal Roll and Flutter.

Before attempting the standard Abdominal Roll it is advisable that you practice with the deep breathing method but do not attempt this method more than four times, as anyone who is not used to using the diaphragm when breathing may find they hyperventilate.

(i)   Assume starting position, with feet slightly apart and knees flexed.

(ii)   Exhale and push your stomach out, then just let it relax.

(ii)   As you inhale slowly, pull your stomach in, imagining that you are trying to touch your spine with it.

(iii)   Then pull your stomach up and hold this position for a minute.

(iv)   Exhale slowly as you push your stomach out, completing an Abdominal Roll.

(v)   Relax then try another before moving on to try this again but this time breathing naturally rather than taking especially deep breaths.

The Abdominal Flutter operates in much the same fashion but a little more simply, so that you just push the stomach in and out rather than rolling it. It can be performed either by breathing gently and naturally or by inhaling and holding your breath. Regardless of the breathing pattern you adopt, however, it should be performed repeatedly and as quickly as possible, keeping in time to the music throughout.

Routines

For those of you who have persevered to the point of feeling confident about both the basic and the advanced moves so far covered, to round up this practical introduction to belly dance I am going to set out some suggestions for routines you might like to try. The guidelines here may need to be adapted so that they fit the rhythm and tempo of whatever music you are dancing to, for example you may find you have to take four forward step-back-steps instead of two or include eight hip-drops-travelling-back instead of four, depending on the length of the section of music you are using.

Routine 1

(i)   Assume start position.

(ii)   Start with eight shimmying hip twists forward on the balls of both feet.

(iii)   Follow this with two forward step-back-steps on the right foot.

(iv)   Then do four hip pushes to the right, then four hips pushes to the left.

(v)   Followed by eight pivoting hip pushes turning to the left.

(v)   Stepping back onto the flat of the right foot do four double hip drops travelling backwards.

(vi)   With four pivoting double hip drops turning to the left.

(vii)   Then four pivoting double hip drops turning to the right.

(viii) Followed by four forward step back steps with shimmy on the spot.

(ix)   Four camel rocks to the right.

(x)   Four camel rocks to the left.

(xi)   Four camel rocks turning to the right.

(xii)   Four camel rocks turning to the left.

(xiii) Then one step and turn step to the right with hip bounce.

(xiv)   Then one step-and-turn-step to the left with hip bounce.

(xv)   Finish up with a spin to the count of eight.

Routine 2

(i)   Assume start position.

(ii)   Place your right leg forward and do four hip rolls with right hip.

(ii)   Follow this with one very large and very slow hip roll before two small undulating hip rolls.

(iii)   Next do one circle within a circle to face the front followed by an upper torso circle.

(iv)   Then four figure eights.

(vi)   Then do two camel rocks to the right followed by two to the left.

(vii)   Raise yourself up onto the balls of your feet and do eight camel rocks turning on the spot to the right.

(viii) Do one slow hip roll (pushing the hips back from right to left) to a count of eight, followed by a hip rotation in the opposite direction.

(ix)   Now sixteen hip twists round in a large circle to the right until you are facing the front.

(x)   Now spin to the right to the count of eight, before spinning to the left, also to a count of eight.

(xi)   Follow this with another sixteen hip twists to the left until you are facing the front and finish off with a spin to the count of eight.

You can now consider yourself to be a fully-fledged belly dancer! However, there are a number of further routines and steps you can learn. The best way to achieve this is to join a local belly dance instruction class for help and guidance and ideas from both teachers and students alike – enjoy!

Bibliography

Aldred, Cyril, *Jewels of the Pharaohs*, New York, Praeger Publishers, 1971

Badger, R, *Great A Fair: The World's Columbian Exposition and Culture*, Chicago, Chicago University Press, 1979

Baigent, Michael, *Ancient Traces*, London, Penguin Books, 1998

Baring, Anne and Cashford, Jules, *The Myth of the Goddess*, London, Arkana, 1991

Benedict, Ruth, *Patterns of Culture,* London, Saqi Books, 1989

Borrow, George, *The Zincali: An Account of The Gypsies of Spain, 1803-1881*

Bounaventura, Wendy, *Serpent of the Nile*, New York, Interlink Books, 1994 and *Belly Dancing: The Serpent and the Sphinx*, London, Virago, 1983

Breasted, James Henry, *Ancient Records of Egypt,* 1906 and *Ancient Times: A History of the Early World*, Chicago, University of Chicago Press, 1916

Burton, Richard Francis, *The Book of a Thousand and One Nights*, Stoke Newington, Benares Kamashastra Society, 1850

Campbell, Joseph, *The Inner Reaches of Outer Space*, London, HarperCollins Publishers, 1986

Carlton, Donna, *Looking for Little Egypt*, Bloomington, International Dance Discovery Books, 1995

Critchfield, Richard, *Shakhat: An Egyptian*, New York, Syracuse University Press, 1990

Croutier, Alev Lytle, *Harem: The World Behind the Veil*, New York, Aberville Press 1989

Crystal, David (ed), *Cambridge Biographical Encyclopaedia*, Cambridge, Cambridge University Press, 1998

Curtis, George Williams et al, *Nile Notes of a Howadji,* New York, Harper and Brothers, 1852

David, Rosalie, *Religion and Magic in Ancient Egypt*, London, Penguin Books, 2002

Denon, Baron Dominique Vivant Denon, *A Journey to Upper and Lower Egypt*, mid 19th century

Durin-Robertson, Lawrence, *The Goddesses of Chaldea*, Eire, Cesara Publications,1975

Eliade, Mircea, *Shamanism: Archaic Techniques of Ecstasy*, Princeton, Princeton University Press, 1951

Flaubert, Gustave, *Travels in Egypt*, 1850

Frazer, Sir James George, *The Illustrated Golden Bough: A Study in Magic and Religion*, New York, Macmillan, 1935

Getty, Adele, *Mother of Living Nature*, London, Thames and Hudson, 1990

Goodwin, Jan, *Price of Honour: Muslim Women Lift the Veil of Silence on the Islamic World*, London, Warner Books, 1994

Gordon-Duff, Lady Lucie, *Letters from Egypt 1862-1869*, London, Routlege and K. Paul,1969

Graves, Robert, *Greek Myths*, London, Penguin, 1955

Haufax, Joan, *The Shaman: The Wounded Healer*, New York, Crossroad/Herder and Herder, 1983

Hogg, Gary, *Cannibalism and Human Sacrifice*, New York, Citadel Press, 1966

Jenkins, Jean and Rovsing Olsen, Paul, *Music and Musical Instruments in the World of Islam*, London, World of Islam Festival Publishing Company, 1976

Johnson, Paul, *Ancient Egypt*, London, HarperCollins Publishers, 1999

Kalweit, Holger, *Dreamtime and Inner Space,* Boston, Shambhala Publications, 1984

Kirch, Patrick, *On the Road of the Winds: An Archaeological History of the Pacific Islands*, San Francisco, University of California Press, 2000

Knight, C, *Blood Relations*, New Haven, Yale University Press, 1991

Lane, Edward William, *Manners and Customs of the Modern Egyptians*, 1836

Lexova, Irene, *Ancient Egyptian Dances*, New York, Dance Horizons, 1975

Lissner, Ian, *The Living Past,* London, Jonathan Cape, 1957

Lommel, Andreas, *Primitive Man*, New York, McGraw Hill, 1966

McDowell, Bart, *Gypsy Wanderers of the World*, Washington DC, Washington DC National Geographic Society, 1970

Maclagan, David, *Creation Myths: Man's Introduction to the World*, New York, W.W. Norton and Company, 1977

Manniche, Lise, *Music and Musicians in Ancient Egypt*, London, British Museum Press, 1991

Mellaart, James, *Earliest Civilisations of the East*, London, Thames and Hudson, 1965

Mernissi, Fatima, *Beyond the Veil: Male and Female Dynamics in a Modern Muslim Society*, New York, Scheukman, 1975

Mertz, Barbara, *Temples, Tombs and Hieroglyphs: A Popular History of Ancient Egypt*, New York, P. Bedrick Books, 1990

Mooney, James, *The Ghost-Dance Religion and the Sioux Outbreak of 1890*, Lincoln, University of Nebraska Press, 1992

Montagu, Lady Mary Mortley, *The Complete Letters of Montagu 1917*, Oxford, Clarenden Press, 1965

Morton, H.V., *Middle East,* London, Methlien and Co Ltd, 1945 and *In the Steps of St Paul*, New York, Myers FHW, 1936

Murnane, William J., *The Penguin Guide to Ancient Egypt*, London, Penguin Books, 1983

Nerval, Gerard de, *Journey to the Orient*, London, Immel Publishing, 1998

Niebuhr, C., *Travels Through Arabia and Other Countries of the East*, Reading, Garnet Publishing,1994

Nieukwerk, Karin Van, *A Trade Like Any Other*, Austin, University of Texas Press, 1995

Osterley, W.O.E., *The Sacred Dance*, Cambridge, Cambridge University Press, 1923

Penzer, N.M., *The Harem*, London, Spring Books, 1936

Plumley, Gwendolen, *The Sudanese Lyre or the Nubian Kissar*, Cambridge, Cambridge Town and Gown Press, 1976

Ranson, Philip, *Tantra: The Indian Cult of Ecstasy*, New York, Crown Publishing, 1988

Redmond, Layne, *When the Drummers Were Women*, New York, Crown Publishing Group, 1997

Ribera, Julian, *Music in Ancient Arabia and Spain: Being La Musica de Las Canticas*, New York, DeCapo Press, 1970

Rippon, Hugh, *Discovering English Folk Dance*, Buckinghamshire, Shire Publications, 1975.

Rogozin, Z.A., *The Nations of the World*, London, Fisher Unwin, 1887

Rudgely, Richard, *Secrets of the Stone Age*, London, Random House Group, 1988

Saadawi, Nawal el, *The Hidden Face of Eve,* London, Zed Books, 1980

Sachs, Curt, *World History of the Dance*, New York, W.W. Norton & Company, 1937 and *The History of Musical Instruments*, New York, W.W. Norton & Company, 1940

Savery, Savery M., *Letters on Egypt*, 1787

Shaw, Ian, *Oxford History of Ancient Egypt*, Oxford University Press, 2000

Shaw, Ian and Nicholson, Paul, *British Museum Dictionary of Ancient Egypt*, London, Harry N. Abrams, 1995

Sjoo, Monica and Mor, Barbara, *The Great Cosmic Mother*, San Francisco, Harper San Francisco, 1991

Stevenson Smith, William, *The Art and Architecture of Ancient Egypt,* New Haven, Yale University Press, 1981

Strouhal, Eugen, *The Lives of the Ancient Egyptians*, Norman, University of Oklahoma Press, 1992

Vitebsky, Piers, *The Shaman*, London, Little Brown, 1995

Wallis Budge, Sir Ernest Alfred Thompson, *The Dwellers of the Nile: The Life, History, Religion and Literature of Ancient Egypt*, New York, Dover Publications, 1926

Watterson, Barbara, *Women of Ancient Egypt*, Stroud, Allan Sutton Publishing, 1998

Westermarck, Edward, *Marriage Ceremonies in Morocco*, London, 1914

Wild, Henry, *Les Danse Sacrees de L'Egypt*, Paris, 1963

Wilkinson, J. Gardiner, *The Ancient Egyptians: Their Life and Customs*, London, John Murray, 1853

Wilkinson, Richard H., *Complete Temples of Ancient Egypt*, London, Thames and Hudson, 2000

Williams Beaumont, Cyril, *Impressions of the Spanish Dancers*, London, A&C Black, 1952

Young, William Charles, *Rashaayda Bedouin: Arab Pastoralists of Eastern Sudan*, Texas, Harcourt and Bruce College Publishers, 1995

Acknowledgements

I am especially indebtd to the following people, without their invaluable help and knowledge this book would not have been possible:

My mentor Caroline Varga Dinicu (otherwise known as 'Morocco') expert on Middle Eastern dance; archaeologists and ancient historians Diane L. Holmes, BA and Nicole Mostafa, BA; Middle Eastern musicians Hossam Ramzy and Russel Harris and the many dancers and musicians I met on my travels while researching for this book; physiotherapists Monique Ellis, SRP and Anne Hawes who expanded my knowledge on physiology and anatomy.

I would also like to thank my family, friends and students for all their support and encouragement.

Thierry Paquot
The Art of the Siesta

Translated by **Ken Hollings**

The Art of the Siesta is a series of vignettes on the importance of the siesta in paintings, literature and sculpture. In *Preliminary*, we hear of the rhythm of sleep, including the fear babies have of going to sleep. In *The Midday Demon,* death in life and erotic dreams take form. The last vignette, *The Siesta Fights Back,* shows how the economic necessities of Western society are conquering the siesta. This is a translation from the French of a book that reinstates the value of sleep in waking hours. From mosques, where guards sleep under the protection of Allah, to 'slow-food' restaurants in Berlin in 2001, it explores the part sleep plays in the cycle of human life.

Thierry Paquot is Professor of Architecture at Paris-la Défense. He is the author of many books, including *Utopia, The Improbable Philosophy of Art, The World of Towns* and a study on Le Corbusier.

£8.95 / $13.95   **ISBN 0-7145-3092-1**

Jean Cocteau
The Art of Cinema

Translated by **Robin Buss**

For more than 30 years, Jean Cocteau maintained a passionate affair with the moving image. To him, film was a visionary dream-like medium, a glimpse of the phantoms that haunted the poet throughout his life. This posthumous collection of writings illuminates Cocteau's work for the cinema, with detailed discussions of his aims, responses to criticism and his reflections on the relationship between poetry, theatre and film. He also comments on the movie stars he admires – Marlene Dietrich, James Dean, Brigitte Bardot – together with such great directors as Georges Franju, Charlie Chaplin and Orson Welles.

Born in France in 1889, **Jean Cocteau** was a visionary poet, film-maker and artist. His films include the avant-garde masterpiece *The Blood of the Poet* and his later meditation on art and mortality, *The Testament of Orpheus*, both published by Marion Boyars as *Two Screenplays*. He died in 1963.

'Extremely discriminating, witty and astute' *The Times*

£9.95/$17.95   ISBN 0-7145-2974-5

Georges Bataille
Literature and Evil

Translated by **Alastair Hamilton**

'Literature is not innocent,' Bataille declares in the preface to this unique collection of literary profiles. 'It is guilty and should admit itself so.' Only through acknowledging its complicity with the knowledge of evil can literature communicate fully. Bataille explores this idea through a series of remarkable studies on the work of eight outstanding authors: Emily Bronte, Baudelaire, Blake, Michelet, Kafka, Proust, Genêt and De Sade.

Born in 1897, **Georges Bataille** was a philosopher, novelist and critic who wrote on a wide range of topics, including eroticism, religion, anthropology and art. Even after his death in 1962, he continued to exert an increasingly vital influence on today's literature and thought. Other works by Georges Bataille available from Marion Boyars Publishers include *Blue of Noon, My Mother, Madame Edwarda and The Dead Man* and *L'Abbe C.*

'Bataille intellectualizes the erotic, as he eroticizes the intellect... reading him can be a disturbing kind of game' *The New York Times*

£10.95/$14.95   ISBN: 0-7145-0346-0

Julian Green
Paris

An American born in Paris at the turn of the last century, Green accompanies the reader on an imaginative stroll around the French capital, revealing its secret stairways, courtyards and alleys and sharing his discoveries at every turn. From haunted visions of Notre Dame to memories of the old Trocadero, Green lovingly describes these strange and often little-known locations.

This special bi-lingual edition is illustrated with the author's own photographs and reveals the hidden delights of Paris in an intimate literary portrait.

Julian Green published over 70 books in France and was a member both of the Académie Française and the American Academy of Arts and Sciences.

'A series of love notes, subtle and charming' *Kirkus*

'Exquisitely literary in a traditional French manner'
New York Review of Books

'you care for good writing and are interested in seeing Paris from
unusual perspective, then try this lovely and elegant book'
ay Times

£9.95/$14.95   **ISBN 0-7145-2928-1**